# WHOLISTIC HEALTH

# WHOLISTIC HEALTH

*A Whole-Person Approach to Primary Health Care*

**Donald A. Tubesing, M.Div., Ph.D.**
*Director, The Institute for Whole Person Health Care,*
*Duluth, Minn.*

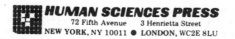
**HUMAN SCIENCES PRESS**
72 Fifth Avenue     3 Henrietta Street
NEW YORK, NY 10011 ● LONDON, WC2E 8LU

Library of Congress Catalog Number

ISBN:0-87705-370-7

Printed in the United States of America
9 987654321

All publications of the Society For Wholistic Medicine can be obtained through:
Wholistic Health Centers, Inc.
137 South Garfield Ave.
Hinsdale, Ill. 60521

**Library of Congress Cataloging in Publication Data**
Main entry under title:

Tubesing, Donald A
    Wholistic health.

    References: p. 223
    Includes index.
    1. Medicine—Philosophy.  2. Family medicine.
3. Pastoral medicine.  4. Wholistic Health Centers,
inc.  5. Medical care—United States.  I. Title.
R723.T84      362.1      78-3466
ISBN 0-87705-370-7

With gratitude to my parents, Murtle, a devoted mother, and Karl, a visionary health care provider ahead of his time, who contributed the most to my health and to my understanding of health care issues.

# CONTENTS

# FOREWORD

As I was reading Don Tubesing's manuscript, I found my-self wondering, "Where did all these interesting insights into health care come from? We certainly didn't have very many of these concepts in mind when we opened the first 'wholistic' clinic in Springfield, Ohio, in 1970."

What has happened, of course, is that philosophical concepts grow out of clinical (human) experiences, particu-larly so because we were fortunate to have a number of committed, bright, health care professionals who kept ask-ing meaningful questions of one another and of patients while ministering to the whole person needs of these pa-tients.

Also, when you put doctors' offices in entirely different settings (in churches, of all places!), and when you sur-round doctors with a different mix of professional helpers, the result is new ways of dealing with health problems.

I have frequently been told that 99% of doctors would be unwilling to practice medicine in the wholistic mode. I believe this, so I am looking for the 1% of doctors (the

3000 doctors in America) who are dissatisfied with the way they are now practicing and would like to risk some changes in their methods and philosophy. This book should assist those readers who are wrestling with such problems at least to know that there are now demonstration projects where they can talk with health care professionals who are enjoying exploration in this new setting.

We have been urged to help establish 40 Wholistic Health Centers in the United States and Canada. Many of them will be related to medical schools and teaching hospitals, so that health care professionals can observe these models and know that they are not locked into traditional ways of practicing medicine. There are other choices!

Don Tubesing, who has worked with me in this project for over 4 years, has brought many things together into a coherent whole. He tells the story in a way that graphically depicts the new excitement in the health care field. There is a mild revolution brewing! He shows us:

> We do not have to continue the old ways of trying to help sick people.
>
> There are new and creative people already participating in testing new ways to understand the voice of illness.
>
> The body's cry for help in illness must also be understood for what it really is—the human spirit crying out for fulfillment, meaning, and purpose.
>
> When people in health care overlook the spiritual dimension of illness, they may be missing the essence of the message that illness is trying to convey.

I am confident that this book will stimulate many practitioners to join the wholistic revolution in health care.

Granger E. Westberg

# Preface

American medicine is not dead, nor is it even dying. There are, however, symptoms of disease. At present, for the most part, these symptoms can be pushed to the back of our consciousness and ignored. But they will only continue to get worse. Unless symptoms are attended to and proper treatment is begun, American medicine may be heading for a breakdown of catastrophic proportions.

This book is a call for a redefinition of health and illness in the context of a broader view of life, health, and the quality of life to include the whole person—the mental, emotional, and spiritual sides of life as well as the physical. It is based on the premise that only a redefinition of health care to include the whole person will begin to lead toward solutions to the problems of the health care system. Only a new way of looking at health and illness will help us to correct some of the many ills.

One solution, the Wholistic Health Center project, is the focus in the description of possible action plans and methodologies for whole person health care. The Wholistic Health Centers are church-based, family practice medical care facilities that utilize an interdisciplinary team of physicians, pastoral counselors (ministers trained in counseling), and nurses who together attend to all aspects of an individual's health needs. Emphasizing health education, early examination, and prevention, and specializing in the treatment and care of the whole person, the Wholistic Health Center project is a creative attempt to respond to some of the weaknesses in the present health care system.

This is not an "antidoctor" book; instead, it is a "pro" book. It is a call for a different way of conceptualizing life, health, and health care. It is a book that suggests practical solutions to some of the problems in health care. It is a book that states emphatically that there is much we can do in moving toward positive, workable solutions.

The book is written for people who work within the health care system, both in the medical and in the nonmedical ("auxiliary") helping fields such as counseling, church work, social work, and education. It is written for those who:

- are tired of griping about the ills of the system and would rather spend their time seeking alternative, better ways of helping people to solve their health problems.
- need to find a new, positive, human-oriented way of continuing to practice their profession before they "burn out."
- believe that we must always take the whole person seriously, no matter what the illness, no matter what our "specialty area."
- believe, based on their knowledge of stress-related, life-style illness, that we just can no longer afford to accept the definition that health is singularly a physical

quality, and that health care is simply treatment for a body that is no longer functioning efficiently.

- want to find a wider vision and some better ways for helping people help themselves become more whole.

This book is written for those who are ready to explore some adventuresome, even risky, ideas, and who will have the courage to put them into practice within their own spheres of work.

Donald A. Tubesing

# ACKNOWLEDGMENTS

A book of this sort, which tells the story of an innovative model for primary health care, is based on the shared insight of an entire staff—people who worked to make the principles behind the model come alive. I have put into context the concepts and care methodologies developed over 4 years by the entire Wholistic Health Center staff. Perhaps it is a testimony to the merit of the Wholistic Health Center project that the names of all who have contributed are too numerous to mention. To all of those who have invested their energies, I feel a debt and a sense of gratitude.

The W. K. Kellogg Foundation and its program staff understood the vision and promise in the Wholistic Health Center concept and supplied the funding necessary to test the ideas. Without this innovative and creative foundation and its thoughtful staff, the health care scene would be missing not only the Wholistic Health Center model, but also many other innovations, which collectively show promise of pointing the way to a more healthful world for all its citizens. The W. K. Kellogg Foundation's important role in our society in general, and in this project in particular, deserves recognition.

Granger E. Westberg, project director and originator, and Edward Lichter, Chairman, Department of Preventive Medicine and Community Health, University of Illinois at the Medical Center, Chicago, under whose auspices this project was administered, have supplied the energy and leadership for the development of the Wholistic Health Centers. Granger's insights and creative vision are appreciated, not only within the project, but across the nation. Excerpts from one of his lectures are included in Chapter 3.

Bill Peterson, Pastoral Director of the Hinsdale center, will find his ideas and paragraphs from various memos scattered throughout the book. His keen mind has greatly stimulated my thinking and generated creative expansion of Granger's original vision for the project.

Perhaps every fledgling author needs a guide and source of encouragement when first confronting the publishing world. Bob Cunningham "volunteered" for this role with me, and I've benefited greatly from his encouragement. Sally Strosahl, Hazel Zimner, Norma Martin, Paul Holinger, and Don Balster have been friends, encouragers, and critics during the writing process. Each lent special expertise and extra effort when needed. Each played a part in trying to keep me sane. Most of the time, they succeeded.

Nancy, my wife and the mother of our two children, Philip and Andrew, believed that this book should be good; she therefore forcefully encouraged me through numerous revisions until the topic was finally presented in an organized manner. I hope her belief will be substantiated.

Many people have played a significant part in my life over the past few years. They all deserve recognition, and they are all thanked in my heart.

D. A. T.

## Chapter 1

# THERE'S TROUBLE IN HEALTH CARE

Normally, the health care system treats patients. Let's turn the tables and apply the technique of medical diagnosis to the system itself. What are the symptoms, the diagnosis, the treatment, and the prognosis? Let's make the medical system the patient, and see what kind of shape it's in.

## AN EXAMINATION

If we take a "history and physical" of the systems of American health care, what do we find?

We find signs that all is well. The patient is growing with leaps and bounds, is steady on his/her feet, is learning new information every day, and is quite healthy. At a quick glance, the patient looks strong and vibrant.

But looking more closely, we find that all is not well. There are signs of trouble. The temperature is rising as the heat of more and more pressure builds up internal stress.

Friends and neighbors are beginning to talk, and they're saying that the patient is haughty, won't listen, and is never available. The patient, still on his/her feet, sure is smart, but never seems to have much heart for people any more. There are signs of sickness and trouble.

## AN ENCOUNTER

Listen to what one neighbor says about her encounter.

> *Background.* "We don't use doctors much, so each place we've been we just contact someone; then whether we like him or not, we stay with him, because we're seldom sick anyway. When we moved here 5 years ago the people had left a list of their doctors and dentists on the wall by the phone. We called one and have used him since."
>
> *He's so busy.* "But he's so busy. He doesn't remember us. Each time we go in we start all over. His waiting room is so full, and he just doesn't have time for you. I see six or eight nurse types, then him for a few seconds. Always I have to deal with the nurses. They talk on the phone, give instructions, get you undressed for exam."
>
> *I get no information or feedback.* "I had two expensive tests done, over $50 each. Waited 3 weeks . . . no word. Called his office. Nurse said, 'Oh, I'll have him call you back.' Six days later he called. He said he had tests in front of him . . . all O.K. He was faking it. I'm sure they came back, were okay, and just got put in the file. No reason to call me if nothing's wrong. The trouble was I was waiting and worried, and they didn't see any reason to let me know I was O.K."
>
> *Recent example.* "One year ago I had stomach pains. Called him; he suggested I go to the hospital for tests. I talked to the nurse; then tests came back. It was gall bladder trouble. The nurse made arrangements for me to go into the hospital. I never saw the doctor—all of this was diagnosed and planned over the phone. Just before surgery, after I'd had an initial tranquilizer before the operation, the doctor came by and said, 'Now what was it we discussed with you about the procedures and problems, etc.?' I said, 'We didn't. We have never talked about it. You have never seen me for this problem!' "

"Well, it was major surgery with some complications, but it all turned out okay. When I got finished with it, though, I decided that's enough of that, I'm not going back."

This is happening all over America. People are sick. They look for help, but often have trouble getting it. When they do find medical help, they often encounter treatment that is mechanically superb treatment for their body, but that demeans them as people. If we listen to friends and neighbors, the patient, the American medical system is still functioning, but it shows symptoms of illness.

There's trouble in health care.

We Americans trust our physicians more than any other government or service personnel, including clergy. For the past 10 years the Harris poll has been surveying Americans on their attitudes toward governmental and service agencies. Every year the medical profession has ranked at the top of the list in terms of public confidence in services.

The medical profession still has our confidence. This is as it should be and needs to be. We can give our vote, or even our tax dollars, to a group we don't trust—in fact, most of us have, like it or not—but we can hardly be expected to lay our lives under the surgeon's judgment and knife if we don't trust the surgeon. The technology of American medicine is miraculous, and it deserves great respect.

However, times are changing and, along with the times, our attitudes toward the persons or systems that deliver valuable services in our communities and nation are changing. In 1966 (the first Harris poll on this subject), 72% of the population surveyed indicated confidence in the medical profession as compared to higher education (61%), religion (41%), and the federal executive branch (41%). In the 1973 poll, medicine still led the list, but with only a 57% vote of confidence. Confidence in the federal government had dropped to 19% in the 7-year span.

Public confidence in the medical profession is diminishing, and trouble is brewing. The voice of consumerism, previously turned on American industry, the military, and the federal bureaucracy, is grumbling about medical care. The irritation we may feel about a car that breaks down or the waste of federal paperwork is nothing like the frustration that boils inside us when someone we love is treated poorly, mechanically or, worse, incorrectly when seriously ill.

American medicine is not dead; it's not even dying. There are, however, symptoms of disease. At present, for the most part, these symptoms can be pushed to the back of our consciousness and ignored. But, if ignored, the symptoms will get worse. Unless the signs of disease are attended to and some effective treatment is begun, American medicine may develop an illness of catastrophic proportions.

## YES, THERE'S TROUBLE: THE GLOOM AND DOOM

On the one hand, American medicine is an amazing complex of technology and capacity to heal acute illness. It is unique in history. Technology has continually improved. We've come a long way from the medicine of Hippocrates, Galen, Harvey, Lister, or even Jonas Salk.

On the other hand, the present situation in the American medical system, by many ways of judging what health care is and should be about, is disastrous.

Hospital costs have escalated during the past 15 years, and no slowdown is in sight. Increases of five and in many cases tenfold are not uncommon. Hospital rooms that in 1960 rented for $20-25 per day now rent for $125 per day.

Physician services for a majority of people, especially for the less affluent and those in rural areas, where the need is the greatest, are minimal and at times unavailable.

There is little treatment for stress-related disease, little coordination of services, little health education—little besides technology.

## Little Treatment for Stress-related Disease

Our population is increasingly wracked by new "silent" epidemics, more insidious, or at least less visible, than those of earlier times. These are not contagious diseases (except for VD, a "social disease"), but degenerative diseases. They are sicknesses brought on by life-style.

Epidemics of stress-related disease are killing at a faster and more steadily advancing rate each year. In the past years the onset of heart disease has increased five times (10 times for those under 40 years of age). Cancer, heart disease, and stroke, all related to life-style, account for 70% of our total deaths due to disease. Gastrointestinal difficulties, hypertension, inability to sleep, and the like add to the total bulk of stress-related health problems. It is obvious that most of the major causes of death relate to life-style.

In many ways the life-style of our nation is sick. The pace of change is accelerating.

Vance Packard has called Americans a nation of nomads, able to pack up all our belongings within a few days and "easily" transport them cross-country to another house almost the same as the one we left. As a nation, we have bought the assumption that moving is relatively painless and a part of progress. Since movers will pack full wastebaskets and ashtrays unless told not to, the only things missing at the other end are familiar landmarks, a personal sense of rootedness, and friends with whom we have a history—the most important items in our lives!

The old values are changing. The family structure is disintegrating, and the church is less than a central guiding force for most people.

Probably none of these dynamics should be labeled negative, except for the fact that this total set of cultural forces is causing ill health among thousands of us. There are epidemics of high blood pressure, depression, early heart disease, suicide, and the like. The new plagues resulting from our style of life are not quick killers, as were those in the past; their havoc is tallied slowly. These plagues are politely labeled "degenerative diseases," which is simply a euphemism for the loss in the quality of life and health over a prolonged period of time—no less insidious a loss, no less insidious a disease.

These pressures of life and resultant new forms of illness related to life-style call for a revised methodology of caring for a multitude of current health problems, unique to our society, that are presently in epidemic proportions.

In relation to this cultural condition, modern medicine, because of the overwhelming demand for crisis care and the failure to take seriously a concept of wholeness in health, often fails to provide adequate preventive health care for life-style diseases. Although modern medicine is technically superior to any known throughout history, the neglected aspects of care call for an increase in health education, an increase in care for the early stages of illness, better coordination of care, and the fostering of support communities for patients experiencing stress-related disease.

*Little Coordination of Services*

Who can help with the whole-person problems that involve the pace of life, emotions, social relationships, beliefs, physical health, and intellectual development all in one lump? A family physician? A psychiatrist? A pastor? A social worker? A family therapist?

Too often the answer is, "No one." And so the problems are left hanging and are not responded to as a whole. That's just what has been happening all over America with a wide variety of human health problems that demand a wholistic approach.

How many people just go home and gamely try to struggle through problems by themselves because no one will listen to the whole story? How many people just go home and live with a problem for 2, or 8, or 25 years because they once tried to get help, got none, and figured, "Well, it's something no one, including me, can do anything about anyway."

The tragedy is that in many cases this simply need not happen. Problems that involve the whole person, which have many disjointed pieces connected only by the history and wholeness of the person who lives with them, can be treated if the whole person instead of the separate problems is given attention.

Specialization now demands that the sick go from one "healer" to another—one for each organ, one for each aspect of illness—searching for answers, trying to understand the information supplied by superspecialists who don't seem to relate to one other, trying to find the key for reducing the pain in their lives, trying to regain a desired measure of health in their lives. Little care is available that focuses on the whole person, the whole context of life, the whole of what it means to be healthy or sick. Resources for health are dispersed in isolation from each other in widely distant centers run by separate disciplines.

## Little Health Education Available

The situation in terms of "health" care is even more disastrous. The present system is sick partly because it focuses almost exclusively on sickness and doesn't marshal its resources for health care. People can get the best, most powerful, and highly concentrated services only after they get sick.

Today there is an almost universal cry for the inclusion of preventive and educational services in the health care system. A significant number of individuals fail to make use of the technical health services available to them. They delay in the face of warning signs and symptoms, they fail to comply with the physician's recommendation for treatment, and they neglect routine preventive examinations. The preventive and health-related activities at the primary level depend almost exclusively on education in order to change behavior.

But, in spite of this, and the obvious need, almost no health education to speak of is done within the context of ambulatory health service centers. Physicians intended to do health education, but they've gotten too busy with crisis care. Health maintenance organizations (HMOs) have planned to include a wide array of preventive and educational services in their package, but to a great extent they have not accomplished what they were designed to accomplish. Presently, most of their health education programming is a response to the federal requirements that an HMO offer health education to its participants. Today most of the traffic in HMOs is really crisis care and, with the second generation of staff and budget analysts taking charge, crisis care, which really pays, is remaining, and the "luxuries" of preventive services are considered secondary.

Health education is a disaster. Out of the national health dollar, 94¢ goes toward the treatment of disease, 4¢ to research, and 2¢ to preventive medicine, of which .4¢ is to health education (Belsky & Gross, 1975). When we consider that most of that .4¢ is spent on information dispensing instead of behavior change, in spite of the fact that the primary causes of many diseases have their roots in people's life-styles and health behaviors, the situation is even worse than disastrous.

Earl Ubel, advocate of preventive medicine and health education, concludes that the challenge to the health care professions is to become a union of educators, not just repairpersons.

> It appears that the lifestyle of populations has as much to do with health as the medical care delivery systems. Diet, exercise, smoking, drugs, accidents, and cleanliness—all related to health—are functions of styles of behavior. Today, the health worker must be as concerned with behavior change leading to health as he is with the delivery of disease care. (Ubell, 1972)

These calls to action are for all practical purposes being ignored. Dentists have been able to sell the idea of prevention and care for the health of the teeth. No other health profession has done nearly as well. Little effort, beyond an occasional inspirational speech, is happening in health education within outpatient settings; still less of what is happening is aimed at behavior changes, and what is happening there hasn't been terribly effective.

There are a lot of good reasons for this. Providers are too busy with crisis care. Patients are afraid to look at their health, afraid they will find something wrong. Patients are unwilling to pay the cost of preventive education while they're still healthy. They aren't used to taking care of themselves and their health, so they tend to ignore small problems until they get really sick; then they request help. Crisis care pays—preventive care does not!

*Little Besides Technology*

Little besides costly surgical remedies designed to correct the destructive effects of disease on the physical organs—

after the damage has occurred—has been developed. Even the supertechnology, as surprising and shocking as this fact may be, has not given evidence that it produces a significantly better chance of helping us live longer or more healthy lives.

Something is wrong. The system is based on what Victor Fuchs calls the "technological imperative"; this is the tendency to do in medicine anything that is technologically possible to do, without weighing the benefits against the cost. This technology-worshipping system is not making and keeping us healthy.

A while back, Thomas Edison dreamed of the future. "The physician of the future," he said, "will give no medicine, but will interest patients in the care of the human frame, in nutrition, and in causes and prevention of illness." Edison's prophecy has not yet become a reality.

Critics and supporters of the present system, including the American Medical Association, Blue Cross-Blue Shield on the one hand, radical consumer groups and California "holistic" practitioners on the other, although professing to disagree with each other and even engaging in professionally veiled forms of hostility and discounting each other openly, agree on one essential point: the present trends must be stopped or the system of health care as we know it in America will topple of its own weight.

Agreeing that something must change is a place to start.

*Our System in Perspective*

Those who have either dabbled in, or concentrated on, wisdom from other cultures and other ages (the collected human wisdom on how health and disease relates to life, culture and relationships), and those who have taken the spiritual view of life and personhood seriously, know that the present American system that we take so for granted as superior, as natural, as the only way is a modern phenomenon, a Western phenomenon, a specifically twentieth-century American phenomenon. No other culture, at no other time in history, has approached illness and its treatment in such a mechanical, scientific, piecemeal, and divided manner.

Perhaps our wisdom is not as superior as we would like to imagine. There are modern examples of countries such as Canada, China, and Sweden that indicate some possible alternate systems for the delivery of health care. Ours is not the only way.

## Gloom and Doom: Concluding Comments

The present situation in the American health care system —judged by almost any standard—is becoming disastrous. There are many good things in the technological prowess and the capability of modern medical science (which is astounding). Physicians, nurses, and hospital administrators are caring, sensitive people. There is much in the present medical armature that is fantastic. (I personally owe technology much for "saving" or at least prolonging the lives of at least two members of my immediate family.) Some of the most dedicated people in the world are working in the medical field. However, the shaky condition of the American health care system may require a revision of the system unless some sense of balance is regained, and human-oriented, whole-person care is restored to its proper place as a top priority, and the focus for care is again put on the whole patient.

## WHAT'S THE TROUBLE?

In the search for a diagnosis, we'll look at the "patient" (the health care system) from a number of viewpoints.

*Complaints of Consumers and Providers*

Everyone has gripes, which indicates that needs are not being met (see Chapter 2). Some books have cataloged these gripes and turned them into best-sellers. That is not what this book is about.

*The System's Inadequacies*

People who look at the problem in depth almost all agree that the "system" is not working smoothly. Individuals (patients and providers alike) are caught in a bind; the system is not delivering quality care to all of our population at a price that they (or even our nation) can afford to sustain. The priorities are out of order, leading to a clumsy allocation of resources (see Chapter 3). Some books call for the destruction of or change within the system. This is not one of those books.

*A Faulty Mindset*

Underneath the gripes and the inadequacies and incapabilities of the system to deliver quality care to all, underneath these "problems," which are symptoms, is the real basis of the sickness: the definition of illness and health, health care, and treatment of disease, as accepted in our culture, practiced by our system of medicine, and adopted by our people, is inadequate. Our way of thinking about our health needs revision (see Chapter 4). This book calls for some redefinition of our concepts of health and health care.

## BEYOND GLOOM AND DOOM

A rash (almost a literary genre) of health books have been published in the past 5 years critizing the system, such as

*Medical Nemesis, The End of Medicine, The American Health Care Empire,* and *Great American Medicine Show.*

In a recent editorial letter in the most prestigious medical journal of all, *The New England Journal of Medicine* (February 1976), Ingelfinger, comments, "Let's have no more of these anti-doctor books, let's have some suggestions, let's hear some better ways. . . . (Ingelfinger, 1976)."

So let's look for some answers and some better ways.

*An Overview*

This book calls for a redefinition of health and illness in the context of a broader view of life, health, and the quality of life in order to include the whole person, and the mental, emotional, and spiritual sides of life as well as the physical. Only a redefinition of health care to include the whole person will begin to lead toward solutions to the problems of the health care system; only a new way of looking at health and illness will help us to correct some of the ills.

This book is not an "anti" book, but a "pro" book. It investigates a whole different way of conceptualizing life, health, and health care. It suggests very real solutions to some of our problems. It states emphatically that there is much that we can do, and it offers positive, workable solutions.

It calls for reviewing and redefining illness and the causes and meanings of illness.

It encourages reviewing and redefining health and the way in which healing occurs.

It describes some ways in which these broader, more humanistic concepts can be translated into action within the present system in a way that makes use of the benefits of modern technology, while focusing on the preservation of, respect for, and attention to, the whole person, and the individual's ability to heal himself/herself.

It emphasizes a more humanized and person-oriented health care.

### The Challenge

Most of us who work within the health care system, in any form of helping people with the physical, emotional, or spiritual "pains" of life, are tired of hearing gripes about what is wrong with our system and our ability to help people. Even those of us who consider ourselves "Antisystem," and who enjoy a good gripe session on occasion, would much rather focus on some positive solutions and spend time seeking alternatives, better ways of helping people to solve their health problems. Sometimes maybe we gripe instead because we fear that no better ways can be found.

It's silly to continue the gripes when there is much each of us can do!

We must return to a more whole-person form of care.

We must always take the whole person seriously, no matter what the illness, no matter what our "specialty area."

We can no longer afford to accept the definition that health is singularly a physical quality and that health care is treatment for a body that is no longer functioning well.

Nobody can really be helped back to full health with that limited approach. We must stop thinking of health care in those terms if we want to be more helpful to others and more enthused about our work.

Most health care people will agree with the need to broaden our view of illness and treatment for disease, with the concepts presented, and with the challenge to develop a more whole-person approach to health care. But some will say, "These ideas are nice, and are probably true, but they're impractical. There's no way I can take the time to put them into practice."

What can we do—each of us in our own little sphere? How can we apply wholistic principles and make them work for the benefit of both patients and providers? There must be many ways. The Wholistic Health Center described in Chapters 5-11 is one way that fits within the system, is paying for itself, and has been received well by the paying sector of the community. It is one project that has sought and found new methods for delivering a more wholistic form of care to people in the early stages of illness. The exact model may not be appropriate for all providers. There are many providers for whom the Wholistic Health Center model would not be possible. For every provider (physician, nurse, dentist, clergy, psychologist, social worker, teacher, etc.) in any setting, however, the principles of the whole-person approach and some of the practical methodologies described in this book as part of the Wholistic Health Center approach can be applied for the greater wellbeing of both the patient and the provider.

This book will bring a message of hope and will stimulate a wider vision of the possible. Instead of being repetitiously critical, it will offer the challenge to become more fully human, more fully humanistic. The invitation is clear. Let us together look for ways to help people help themselves become more whole.

## Chapter 2

# EVERYONE IS DISSATISFIED WITH THE QUALITY OF HEALTH CARE

## EVERYBODY HAS GRIPES—THESE GRIPES EXPRESS NEEDS THAT ARE NOT BEING MET

To ask "What's the trouble?" is not a neutral beginning. This question is asked when there are clear signs that something is wrong. Most often a physician, member of the clergy, counselor, teacher, relative, or friend will ask a person "What's the trouble?" when it's obvious that something is wrong, but exactly what is wrong is not clear.

That's the situation in American health care today. It's obvious that something is wrong, but exactly what is wrong is not clear.

What is the problem? Where does the trouble lie? It's not hard to find diagnosticians who have answers to these questions. Patients, physicians, clergy, psychologists, social workers, nurses, and legislators each have their own answer, which amounts to a diagnosis based on the symptoms of the system they experience when approaching it from the perspective of their own needs.

Everyone, it seems, is frustrated, perhaps even angry. Patients and providers all have complaints. These complaints indirectly express some very real personal needs that are not being met by the present health care system. Everyone has picked some handy personal target on which to unload the blame.

Hidden within these complaints are some honest answers to the question "What's the trouble?" and some helpful indication of changes that are needed.

## THE PATIENT'S VIEW

I work as a pastoral counselor in a medical setting. Whenever and wherever I meet new people, when they hear about my involvement with the wholistic approach to health care, they invariably begin sharing some personal story of hurt, distrust, bitterness, and anger at the way they have been treated.

One of the occupational hazards of my association with the Wholistic Health Centers is my unsolicited role as "wailing wall" for the dissatisfied consumer of health care services.

The kinds of conversations I've had over the past few years have highlighted a number of areas about which consumers consistently gripe. These gripes are sometimes accurate and justified, and are sometimes distorted. Their significance, however, is found in the definition they provide of the problems in American medicine as seen by the patient.

Running through these problems is an undertone of criticism of the private physician. This is not surprising, since for most people their "health care action" takes place in the physician's office; 80% of health care visits are to private physicians. The physician, therefore, is most often defined by the consumers as the target for the negative feelings they experience when their needs are not fully met.

And so patients say "The trouble is. . . ."

*The Trouble Is . . . Long Waiting Times at the Doctor's Office*

> "I hate waiting in a waiting room and then an examining
> room for 1-1/2 hours and then only being seen by the doctor
> for 5 minutes."
> "I have waited 1-1/2 hours (or longer) after the scheduled
> appointment time in the pediatrician's office. Although I
> sympathize with them for trying to see sick children (I want
> my sick child seen!), I feel rushed when I finally do see the
> doctor, guilty about taking her time when she's so busy, and
> forget things I need to ask."
> "In O.B.-Gyn. I know the schedule is hectic, but more cour-
> tesy would be nice, especially when I have to take little kids
> along. Sometimes I have waited 2–3 hours."

Patients resent the long waiting periods, but seem to
accept them as part of the price that must be paid in order
to see the doctor. The feeling of being rushed once they do
get to see the doctor is common. Some people make lists
of questions on note cards so that they won't forget important items during the few rushed minutes with the physician.

The nonverbal message of 2–3 hour waits is clear:
"Your time is not important—the doctor's time is important." Polite and considerate human relationships would
dictate that when a 2–3 hour delay is expected because of
an unavoidable emergency, the patient should be told, and
invited to stay or go shopping and run errands in the mean-
time.

*The Trouble Is . . . Doctors Are Not Available When I Need
Them*

> "I can tell when I'm sick. Unfortunately, the office nurse has
> to agree with my decision before I can see the doctor."
> "It's too much red tape to get in."
> "I believe the greatest problem the health care system has
> is overspecialization and too few G.P.s available."

> "There are unreasonable delays in obtaining appointments. One day I suddenly couldn't focus my eyes very well—I couldn't get an appointment for a month. I had to live with the worry, and I received no treatment for the whole month. (The only time you can get an immediate appointment is when somebody at the doctor's office decides you're super-sick.)"
>
> "What should I do when my kids get really sick at night or on weekends?"

The availability of physicians raises a whole spectrum of personal concerns. (1) What do I do after hours in case of an emergency—bother the physician, or go to the emergency room? (2) Why can I get appointments only during hours when I work? (3) It is difficult to remember scheduled appointments made 1 or 2 months earlier; it is even more difficult to guess that far ahead what my schedule will be.

People feel put off, as though they must crash through a wall and be dying to see the physician. Receptionist–nurses often act as "gatekeepers" and won't let patients talk to the doctor. But often they aren't knowledgeable enough to answer questions of immediate concern. Almost everyone knows some qualified young person who couldn't get into an American medical school. "Why is that," they wonder, "when we need more doctors?"

*The Trouble Is . . . Only Crisis Care Is Available*

> "It's such a hassle to get an appointment that I never go unless I simply cannot stand it any longer. Then I call and demand to be seen immediately."
>
> "There's not enough prevention of poor health. I wanted time with the doctor to talk about the growth and nutrition of my children, but I couldn't see him—he was too busy with really sick people."

As a result of the limited availability of physician time, a pattern of responding only to emergencies is developed.

Many physicians want to do preventive care, but often have trouble just staying ahead of the crises. Patients, knowing the difficulties and delays in making an appointment, wait until they're sure that they're really sick before calling.

*The Trouble Is . . . Medical Care Costs Too Much*

> "The charges are out of sight, ridiculous. And I had trouble even getting an itemized bill from the hospital."
> "After my physical, my doctor ordered several more lab tests which he said were not really that necessary, but he routinely orders them to protect himself from malpractice. The extra tests came to $40."

Patients are at the mercy of physicians, laboratories, and hospitals regarding fees. Rarely are they consulted in advance about the cost of procedures, services, drugs, hospitalization, and the like. The treatment is prescribed and carried out, the bill comes as a nonnegotiable shock a week or a month later.

Several factors complicate the problems of high costs.

1.   Most insurance plans won't pay unless people are hospitalized; therefore, many people go into the hospital when it is not necessary. There's a financial reward for being really sick (insurance will pay for it), but not for being relatively healthy and trying to take care of yourself before you get really sick (you pay for that yourself).
2.   When people are dissatisfied with their care, they often resist paying their bills or counter with malpractice suits, thus raising the cost of care.
3.   Modern technology combined with lack of planning for areawide health services has resulted in a proliferation of seldom used, very costly technical equipment in each hospital. Competition instead of interinstitutional cooperation has thus resulted in high overhead costs, eventually borne by the patient.

## The Trouble Is . . . Doctors Don't Do Their Homework on Patients

"No doctor has ever asked to have my old (family) records transferred to him. It takes a few years for records to get completed and up-to-date in his office, and then we move; the records never catch up with with us."

"I twice phoned my gynecologist for a tranquilizer prescription. He spent quite a while on the phone with me. When I came for a routine checkup several months later, he had no recall and no record of my problem or his prescription. I question: Is it lack of interest? Doesn't he care? Or does he just keep poor records?"

"After my child had bronchitis the doctor took an X ray. Thirty-six hours later he finally called back with the information that my child had pneumonia."

"My pediatrician's partner phoned to give my son a prescription for penicillin because his strep culture was positive. I had to ask questions and inform him that my son had been on a 30-day maintenance dosage already. He just called with the lab results—he didn't even pull the chart and read it."

Undoubtedly both overwork and lack of interest in keeping good records contribute to the poor system of communication. Lab tests are stuck in files and patients never get called, as though the doctor and not the patient rightfully "owned the information." Personal health records aren't passed from one doctor to another. Two or three specialists may be treating the same individual with noncompatible medication without knowing it. The best check on error (the patient) often keeps his/her mouth shut and doesn't raise enough questions to point out the error.

## The Trouble Is . . . Mechanized, Impersonal Care

"Our doctor has become overworked and has lost his personal touch. We were one of the first patients of a new doctor in a big clinic—our first physical (husband and wife).

The doctor was very relaxed, personable, thorough, and seemed to care. On each subsequent visit or phone call, he has become more and more brusque, abrupt, and 'hassled.' Both the doctor and the patients have lost the original good rapport."

"I took my two children (ages 7 and 9) to the pediatrician for a routine physical. The doctor never spoke to the children except to tweet, chirp, whistle, or joke. All serious conversation was carried on over their heads with Mother. The children felt they had been treated as infants and refused to see that doctor again."

"The office is too mechanized—patients are called from the waiting room by a loudspeaker system. Doors are opened by buzzers. The staff is so segregated from the patients that I wondered, 'Is anybody there?' "

"The specialists I've gone to recognize me only when they have my name in front of them."

People do indeed notice that the closeness, warmth, and personal history once characteristic of the relationship with their G.P. is now missing. They resent being treated like a "thing" that falls into a specific category because of what seems to be a specific medical problem. Phrases such as "I'm a number," "I feel like I'm wasting his VALUABLE time" and "He's so busy," indicate that the loss of a personal touch is noticed. Women notice that most doctors are men, and many feel they are treated in a demeaning way because they are women.

These charges may or may not be accurate. The feelings, however, are real and probably stem to a great degree from the impersonal, mechanical, hurried care experienced in many offices.

A number of factors contribute to the feeling that care is mechanical. The sense of a defined patient group for which a physician is personally responsible is lessening as patients become more dispersed, less identifiable as a group, and use specialists directly without referral.

The importance of high-quality medical care based on scientific and technological excellence is generally accepted by patients. "In addition, what they often want, however (but do not state), is someone who cares, who relieves anxiety, who provides some support through the pain and turmoil of life, and who gives advice and help as well as 'scientific ministrations.' " (Andreopoulos, 1974)

*The Trouble Is . . . I Get Treated Like a Child*

> "I'm never asked about the prescription or treatment. It's just, 'Here's what you must do.' "
> "Doctors generally will not explain findings, medications, etc., unless I pin them down. Their general attitude has been, 'You wouldn't understand; just do as I say.' "
> "I find out now that 10 years ago my dentist merely 'patched up' my teeth, rather than describing an alternative treatment that would have saved more teeth. He never mentioned an alternative to me. When I confronted him last winter he said, 'Oh, I didn't think you were ready for that, or had the money.' It should have been my choice."
> "No one told me what to expect either before or after surgery, just that 'it had to be done.' "

Problems that arise from people being treated (and thus acting like) irresponsible children include: (1) patients don't get to tell the doctor everything they know about their condition; (2) medications are dispersed without information on their side effects or interactions; (3) the doctors make some judgments and decisions that rightfully should be made only by the individual affected; and (4) patients often don't cooperate with or subtly resist the treatment and procedures.

Counselors, dentists, and hospital personnel all receive the criticism that they keep the patient in the dark. One hospital outpatient education program taught people to take their own blood pressure. When a graduate of that program entered the same hospital, he was told by the nurse that she could not tell him his temperature and blood pressure. The mystique that the patient cannot understand

and has no right to know is an appropriate focal target of activated consumers. Patients are ready and able to take care of themselves.

*The Trouble Is . . . My Doctor Is Interested Only in My Body*

"I clearly remember the day I was diagnosed as an adult diabetic. The doctor looked at my lab test results (I hadn't slept well the night before while waiting), and he said, 'You're definitely diabetic. I want you to start on insulin. Come back tomorrow and we'll teach you to start injections and make an appointment with the nutritionist.' With that he escorted me out of the office. (The subsequent educational session took place through a haze of grief, which no one asked or warned me about.) After 2 years I am finally beginning to accept the disease and make decisions to take care of myself. I asked the doctor whether my diabetes could be related to the stress in my life, which was at a crisis point at the onset of the disease. He said it definitely wasn't. A few weeks later he said, 'You may need more insulin when you're under stress.' "

"My life was spared through the miracles of technology, but after the emergency hysterectomy I was told, 'You're lucky to be alive.' I was given a lifetime prescription for estrogen, and sent out to fend for myself. No one helped me through the next years of emotional trauma. No one seemed to care. They felt they had done their job by keeping me alive."

The fact that stress and life-style factors are important components in the development and alleviation of many illnesses has been demonstrated by medical science. For the most part, however, this information is ignored in the diagnosis and treatment, which usually center on symptom descriptions and medication prescription.

If personal values, beliefs, goals, relationships and other aspects important to the quality of life were to be discussed seriously in the doctor's office, too much time would be used up. Physicians prefer to prescribe a pill and set up a return appointment in 2 weeks.

*The Trouble Is . . . Basic Bad Manners and Human
Insensitivity*

> "When I had sexual problems, the doctor brusquely told
> me, 'There's no physical problem—you just don't want to be
> married.' "
> "When I was worried about the wound not healing well and
> not feeling my old self yet, I was simply told, 'Forget it—it's
> nothing to worry about.' "
> " 'Your son is very sick,' he told me. 'It's a good thing you
> have lots of children.' Like as if one death wouldn't matter
> as much then."

People want to be treated as whole persons. All of us
want someone to listen to our feelings and take them seriously. All illness, especially serious illness, generates an
immense variety of feelings and questions, fears, and dis-
couragements. Physicians seem to communicate that
they're too busy to listen. Maybe it's fear. Maybe they have
little training or interest in this side of health care. If so,
then someone who is capable of discussing the impact of
health problems on other dimensions of a person's life
should be enlisted as part of the team.

A great deal of patient experience in medical crises
seems to be described by "technical miracles and human
insensitivity."

## SUMMARY

One patient summarized her feelings by saying, "I'm always left hanging on the phone, right away I'm put on
hold." It's the patient whose welfare ostensibly is the total
and only appropriate focus for the medical care industry.
It's the same patient who is most consistently "put on
hold." Perhaps that action is a symbol of the whole problem as seen by consumers.

One participant in a recent seminar on wholistic health care summed up the needs of the consumer.

> "What I want is to find a physician who gives quality medical care but who will listen to me, and care, and take what I have to say seriously. Goodness knows, I'm not the expert on medicine. I don't want to tell the doctor what to do. That's why I go to him for his ideas and knowledge. But I want to be respected as a human being, and I simply will not accept any longer the old runaround I've gotten before. Although right now I honestly don't know where I can find what I want."

## THE PHYSICIAN'S VIEW

If the patient's complaints and their perceptions of medical care problems were totally accurate, the solution would be easy—change the doctors. The truth, however, is that most health care providers are caught in some of the same dilemmas that the patients' comments highlight.

My role in the development of the Wholistic Health Centers project has also put me in touch with many health care providers, including physicians, nurses, counselors, clergy, educators, and social workers, who also have their gripes about each other and about the people for whom they care.

People in the health care professions are also angry and frustrated. They are angry about the difficulties they experience in finding enough time to spend with people who need their service, angry about being set up as technologists, and resentful about unreasonable demands placed on them by patients who don't want to get well. Many are frustrated by trying to balance their professional responsibilities with living a life that includes caring for the people they love and finding time and energy to spend on their own private life goals and personal interests.

Almost all doctors entered medical school with the intent to serve people. Most practicing physicians are still intent on providing the kind of in-depth caring, combined with technically superior health care, that the patients desire.

Unfortunately, individual doctors, however well intentioned, are caught in a situation that demands compromises. There is simply too much technical information for any one person to master and keep up to date. So they specialize and join specialist teams in a central location. There are too many people who could use the advice and care of the physician, so limits are drawn, and those with the greatest crises get the most attention.

Most consumers act as though they are "crisis oriented," so physicians, hospitals, and insurance plans are also crisis oriented. Most doctors simply aren't trained to "counsel" with people regarding their emotional reactions to illness, the effect of stress on their health, their faith, and their value systems. So they tend to stay away from attention to these life factors and stick with what they know best.

The waiting room fills up. The doctor becomes more harried, impatient, and less receptive to listening carefully to patient concerns. Most physicians recognize that continuous personalized care, coordination of services, and feedback to patients suffer but, in the light of few alternatives, they become resolved to these factors and at times defensive about them.

And so, physicians say, "The trouble is. . . ."

*The Trouble Is . . . I'm Trained as a Medical Doctor, Not a Psychologist*

"Some of my patients would talk for an hour if they ever got started."
"I'm not 'Dear Abby' or a psychiatrist—I'm a medical doctor, and that's what I trained for—recognizing arrhythymias

and aneurisms, not the complicated social-psychological
patterns that I can't do anything about."
"The media is partly to blame. I think health education is
great, but almost every day somebody is in my office con-
vinced they have whatever rare complication is reported in
this month's magazines or last night's TV shows."

Medical schools and residency specialty programs
train physicians in the science of technological medicine.
The course schedules are jammed with enormous quanti-
ties of information that must be mastered. The responsible
physicians attempting to keep up with the latest scientific
knowledge in order to deliver the best possible care for
their patients find the task almost overwhelming.

Even general practice physicians are scientific specialists. This is a result of both personal strengths and professional training. The physician with the patience for
listening to emotional issues and with training in counseling skills is an exception.

*The Trouble Is . . . Patients Are Insensitive, Discourteous*

"Why do some people feel they should have a private pipe-
line to the doctor whenever they decide it's convenient for
them?"
"I get fed up with people who believe no problem is too
trivial to wake me up at 1:00 a.m. if they suddenly decide
they are sick."
"I guess my patients could be divided into three groups.
Those who would bother me with any trivial symptom any
time of the day or night (usually not during office hours);
those who ignore all the symptoms until a major crisis occurs
—maybe too late; and the rare ones who know when to call,
and when to take care of themselves."

The physician-patient interaction forms a relationship.
Every person brings needs for personal fulfillment and self-
respect to any relationship. When health care professionals, especially physicians, are literally running themselves

ragged attempting to respond to the real crisis needs of their patients, the insensitive and hostile demands of a few cannot help but produce feelings of frustration and resentment.

## The Trouble Is . . . Patients Won't Take Care of Themselves

> "What do you expect? I told that Mother, 'absolutely nothing by mouth' for her toddler with vomiting and diarrhea. Then as soon as the kid stopped upchucking for half an hour she's feeding her again—and the whole cycle starts all over again."
>
> "The only way I can be sure the child is taken care of properly is to hospitalize her. Why bother calling me if you're not going to do what I recommend?"
>
> "Patients don't take care of themselves. I told him he had to lose 40 pounds and quit smoking. Now here he is again having gained weight—and still smoking. How can I take care of him?"

People often call on the physicians and hope they can perform miracles. Many people act as if they don't want to be bothered with the responsibility for helping to take care of themselves. In fact, some hope that the physician can come up with some painless remedy that will minimize the negative results of their poor health habits, just so that they can continue to live unhealthy life-styles and get away with it. When patients refuse to take any responsibility for themselves and the condition of their own health, much of the physician's ability to help is undercut.

## The Trouble Is . . . I Don't Have the Time

> "Sometimes I have a list of 20 phone calls to make when I finally get some breathing space in my office hours."
>
> "I'm already running myself ragged between morning hospital calls, and afternoon office hours that often would extend into the evening if I stopped to pay more than cursory attention to my patients."

"I've trained my office nurse to screen out telephone calls and attend to the routine problems herself. If I talked to everyone who calls I'd never get time to see my office patients."

"Insurance forms are a real headache. I hired one person full-time just to do the paperwork."

"My family never sees me. I leave before the kids get up and rarely get home before they go to bed. And once I'm home there's always the telephone with somebody demanding my time."

Health care professionals often don't get the satisfaction out of their profession that they had expected. Some are literally killing themselves in attempts to respond to so many people with so many needs, and to do this in an increasingly complex bureaucratic jungle of paperwork and administrative hassles.

Being a conscientious physician is a complex job. Routinely, physicians will have patients in several different hospitals. In addition to hospital rounds and office hours, the day is eaten up by teaching conferences, consultations, and phone calls from patients and pharmacists. It takes time and emotional energy and an extremely high sense of commitment to do the research and investigation necessary to devise a treatment plan tailored to each individual.

*The Trouble Is . . . It Costs a Lot to Care for People*

"People gripe about high costs—but they never think about how expensive it is to run an office, fill out insurance forms, pay the answering service, the overhead, plus the malpractice insurance."

"Nor do they realize how many people I take care of who either can't afford to pay or don't bother to."

"I'm still trying to pay off all the loans I needed when I was in medical school and starting up practice."

"I could have gone into some soft specialty like radiology or dermatology—where the hours are reasonable and the hassles less."

Running a successful medical practice is big business. It takes a high level of organizational, administrative, and financial skills. In addition, patient crises to which the physician constantly is asked to respond make time for the long-term planning that is necessary for managing such a business very difficult to find. These responsibilities inherent in every medical practice are not visible to or appreciated by most patients.

*The Trouble Is . . . I'm Only Human and People Expect Me To Be God*

> "I'm being sued right now by a former patient for whom I went 'the extra mile,' but since her condition did not fully improve, she's claiming that I am incompetent. That hurts more than my pocketbook."
>
> "People expect me to know all the answers—all the time 'be perfect'—I'm only human, I get tired, make mistakes, sometimes I don't know the answers."
>
> "Medicine is not an exact science—we know some things, but not everything. Somehow I have to find time, energy, and money to keep up with what's happening—even though I can't always know for sure that a particular treatment will work."
>
> "People expect me to remember all their medical problems, and to diagnose and prescribe over the phone."
>
> "People expect miracles. I'm just a doctor."

The demand to be perfect, to play God, is an impossible one for any human being to meet. There is no way physicians can hope to respond to all the multiple and unrealistic expectations placed on them by patients.

## SUMMARY

The enormous increase in technical knowledge, the constant needs of patients for crisis care, the discourteous patients, the unrealistic expectations of patients, and the complexity of managing the business side of the practice add up to a set of demands on the physician's time and emotional energy that are impossible for any one person to fulfill.

In response to the many uncompleted tasks and constant pressures, physicians may begin to feel a nagging sense of failure. Constant demands often produce a phenomenon known nontechnically as "burnout." Symptoms of the disease burnout include: anger and hostility at those making demands; unwillingness to allow others to be close; diminished ability to be warm and intimate; or escape— escape to noncontact pursuits such as research or administration, escape through illness, escape by leaving the profession, escape by concentration on building material wealth and/or exotic, expensive forms of recreation. Generally, these symptoms of burnout are seen by consumers not as symptoms of the pressures on physicians, but as disease itself. Generally, consumers complain about the symptoms instead of being sensitive to the underlying causes.

The complaints of and pressures on providers are not limited to physicians; they apply to health care professionals in general. Psychologists, social workers, clergy, schoolteachers—all are subject to consumer complaints. All have their own lists of complaints about the demands placed on them.

*Patients*

A too-long wait, crowded offices, no time to ask questions, 6 weeks to wait for an appointment, the office is so far away, no one knows my name, the answering service couldn't help, can only get help if I'm dying, it costs too much, they lost the test, no one cares, they treat me like a child, no one listens to my feelings and fears—the list of gripes goes on and on.

Undergirding all the gripes seems to be a sense among patients that they are not respected as human beings. They are consistently treated in ways that in any other business, in any other interpersonal contact, would be labeled unacceptable impoliteness and disrespect. American consumers are unhappy about much of the way they are treated as persons when asking for medical care.

The anger and confusion people feel in the face of the problems they experience with modern medical care are evidenced in numerous ways. Some people stay away. Some people sue. Some people get sicker and don't get the quality kind of health care that should and could be available to them.

*Physicians*

Doctors also feel resentment, anger, and hurt when they are swamped with work and someone pushes them too hard, when they have had too many night calls for the past week, when patient after patient sets them up as "God," when patients simply refuse to hear suggestions on how they must take care of themselves to regain health, when patients gripe about the bills they receive, and when they get hopelessly behind schedule.

There is too much to be done and too little time. Some physicians respond by working so many hours that they "marry" their profession and their families don't know them—or leave them. Others call the limit earlier and shorten their hours. Still others escape to ranches and yachts. Whatever their method of handling the demands, physicians are not the whole cause—so they can't be totally the cure.

Consumers are angry. Doctors are harried and defensive. Other providers, nurses, clergy, counselors are not normally included on the health care team.

The interface between the consumer and the provider

forms a human relationship with some problems that must be faced. As with any relationship, one side is never totally at fault. It takes two to argue, to be angry, to hurt. Continuing in a relationship that is less constructive than it could be, especially when both parties see the necessity and desire to change, is inexcusable. More of the same simply will no longer do. If physicians refuse to allow change in the way they practice, or if patients refuse to change the way they think of their health and relate to their doctors, then either or both will be at fault.

Who is the victim? Who is the cause? The medical profession, in failing to listen to consumers and in resisting almost all change, has helped to create the present chaos. The patients, by the way they both accept and demand crisis-oriented care, also perpetuate the problems. Individual people, both providers and patients, get caught in the cross fire, in a problem that is too big for one patient or one physician to solve successfully.

What's the trouble? It's not hard to find diagnosticians who have answers to this question. Both consumers and providers have some handy targets on which to unload the blame. Everyone has complaints. Behind all the complaints are needs. How can we get behind the complaints, listen to the needs, and move toward responding to these real needs of both providers and patients which are not presently being met?

The following chapters deal further with this question.

## Chapter 3

# THE SYSTEM OF HEALTH CARE DELIVERY IS INEFFICIENT

## MISPLACED PRIORITIES

Americans are not getting a healthy dollar's worth for the health dollar spent. Within the next few years Americans will be spending at least 10% of the total gross national product (GNP) on health care. Presently, the level is 8% and rising. Yet the care available to our citizens is no better (and in some ways is worse) than that in countries that spend half that percentage and far less total dollar amounts. Something is wrong.

Health care professionals are not getting satisfaction out of their professions, either. They are overworking themselves in attempts to help other people and to live in an increasingly bureaucratic jungle. The problem is that health care resources are being utilized primarily as sickness care resources.

## THE SYSTEM IS THE TROUBLE

Something is tragically wrong in the health care delivery system if neither consumers nor providers are getting what they need. Perhaps both patients and physicians are victims of the priorities set by the medical system, which has emphasized the technology of medicine, increasing specialization, and a style of private entrepreneurship instead of the delivery of care to people. Perhaps the system is the problem.

It's possible that a partial answer to the complaints of both patients and providers concerning time, access, cost, and so on, would be a reallocation of health care services to meet the primary care needs of the mainly healthy, occasionally sick majority and not those of the critically ill minority.

### The Medical Care System

One inadequacy of the present health care system is the misallocation of resources. There are not enough personnel focused on primary care and general practice. How, with the expenditure of 8% of the GNP on health care, is this possible? The expenditures are sufficient. The funds, however, have been spent in a disorganized, unplanned manner by governmental and private health, educational, service, and research agencies. The focus has been on the development of technology and specialists instead of on the recruitment and training of person-oriented general practitioners.

At present, our medical care system relies on the availability of private physicians. In 1969, 77.9% of all outpatient primary care visits were made to private practice physicians. Yet the physicians' accessibility is decreasing for three reasons: (1) diminishing numbers, (2) limitation on hours in practice, and (3) the tendency to move away from local neighborhoods and to centralize the medical facilities and offices. This means that physicians are moving away from people, and people are having a more difficult time getting in touch with them (Andreopoulos, 1974).

During the last 40 years the number of general practitioners has been cut in half, while the population has doubled. In 1931 the ratio of general practitioners to the population was 1 per 1060. In 1971 this ratio was 1 to 2430. There are more licensed physicians in our country today than in 1940. However, in 1940, 62% of them were in general practice. In 1970 only 19% were in family or general practice (Andreopoulos, 1974). The system hinges on the availability of physicians, and the physicians simply are not available to the general public in sufficient numbers to respond to the needs of many people. No wonder people are unhappy with the health care available.

The medical care system designed to respond, with enormous technology, to serious acute disease is ill-equipped to respond to the life-style, stress, and degenerative disease issues affecting the quality of our lives as whole persons.

The distribution of health care resources is unequal: the wealthy have plenty, the poor have little; the very sick can get much, the "worried well" get little. Medical education is entrenched in education for supertechnical specialty care instead of personal care. Many private enterprise physicians see 10 patients per hour (6 minutes per patient, on the average). The centralization of services has made care less available and thus more crisis-oriented.

Where is a health care, focused on personal needs of the whole person, in the early stages of illness? For most of us it's a well-kept secret.

*The Mental Health Care Systems*

Of course, medicine is not the only health care system that is out of balance. The priorities within the "auxiliary" health care systems are often disrupted and in internal chaos because of differing ideologies, the competition for funding, and interprofessional jealousy.

For better or for worse, as a society we have defined mental health as a separate and distinct entity.

During the 1840s and 1860s, our country indulged itself in cultural purification rites by building massive state institutions for the mentally insane. Persons whose behavior did not fit the American rationalist dream (i.e., that education of the populace would solve the ills of society) were simply locked up so that the rest of the country would not have to face seeing that their society was not perfect.

Recently the mental health counseling professions have developed into a respected health care speciality. We no longer lock people up with such finality and such regularity. Unfortunately, however, when so little is known about how to help people live responsible, fulfilled lives, the professions, as they have developed, have isolated themselves from each other in order to "fight" for their own acceptability and identity.

There are psychiatrists, social workers, and psychologists (clinical, counseling, social, and other types), and guidance counselors, pastoral counselors, and marriage and family counselors—none of whom like each other very much or accept each other's credentials very readily. There are family service agencies (where a social work degree is required for employment), county mental health clinics, psychiatric wards in the local hospital, and school psychological centers, each generally run separately from other mental health efforts in the area and almost certainly run separately from other types of medical health care efforts.

In the confusion that results from interdisciplinary suspicions, misunderstanding, and ignorance, people are allowed to fall between the cracks without getting the full range of attention most likely to assist them in maintaining or regaining the fullest measure of their health.

## The Institutional Church

Even the religious systems at times seem more intent on self-preservation than on the care of people.

Religious faith is a core dimension of human life. One's belief system is the integrating factor in life. The Judeo-Christian tradition, which forms the basis for most structured religious activity in this country, has at its disposal a powerful message of grace, forgiveness, freedom, and wholeness—a message for health.

However, the churches as institutions have fossilized this message in dogma. They have invested in buildings, not people. They have often organized for efficiency instead of for care; the result is that much of the meaning and power of the message is blunted and the churches' impact is no longer felt by a majority of the populace.

Somehow the churches have become a product of our culture instead of its shaper. The prophetic message has been lost. The volume of the loud, clear call that challenges our cultural signs of unhealth—the hunger for power and material—has been turned down to a nearly inaudible level.

The church has too often limited its role in health care to the "soul," wherever or whatever that may be, and has thus done injustice to the message of personal wholeness necessary for a positive definition of health. Hospital chaplains are usually not really on the health care team, even in church-owned hospitals.

The result is that the positive, powerful message that speaks a word of health to the whole person doesn't sound clearly; and, in the midst of loss of meaning, hopeless feelings, unclear values, apathy, and conformity experienced by many people, they don't sense the relevance of the churches' message, and they turn it off.

Maybe it's the system that's the trouble—the medical care system, the mental health system, the institutional church system.

It seems that in America we have systems designed to offer excellent care for the very sick. The fine-tuned sensitivities and coordination needed for offering care to those who "just don't feel well," however, are mostly undeveloped and unavailable. Our health care systems need to focus efforts on refining their ability to offer quality care to those in the early stages of ill-health before full-blown sickness develops. Our health care systems must learn to coordinate efforts for the good of the patient.

## THE SYSTEM AND STRESS-RELATED ILLNESS: THE THREE ACTS OF ILLNESS*

How do the delivery patterns of the health care system relate to the development of disease in people's lives? Let's look at three progressive stages in the development of stress-related illnesses and examine the resources for health care that are available in each stage. The juxtaposition of these two elements (the resources and the stage of illness) may help to clarify the contention that it's partly the system that's the trouble and needs changing.

### The Development of Illness: Three Acts

Stress-related illness tends to come on gradually as the effects of an unhealthy life-style slowly take their toll. Usually stress-related disease begins with symptoms that are barely noticeable; if the cause remains untreated, the symptoms become more painful and less easy to ignore.

A person who is hospitalized with a stomach ulcer partially caused by stress and pressure first noticed other symptoms such as heartburn, increased stomach gas, and

*The "Three Acts of Illness" is written from notes of an original presentation by Granger E. Westberg.

irregular bowel movements and ignored them until the disease was fully developed and could no longer be ignored. Parents may notice crankiness, tiredness, a pale look, or decreased appetite in their child a day or two before the child complains of a sore throat. Warning signs that indicate that a person is "just a little bit sick" usually generate into more serious symptoms unless the early signs are noted and treated appropriately.

Stress-related illness (often called psychosomatic or functional illness) is a real physical sickness brought on, or magnified by, other life pressures and life-styles. Family physicians tell us that 50–75% of the patients they see in their office have some form of stress-related illness. Some physicians say it's closer to 80–90%. This means that most people who are "a little bit sick" with colds, backaches, headaches, insomnia, and the like, can choose to ignore the symptoms until they get worse, or can choose to change something in their life-styles and behavior patterns before they get sicker. This means that people can do something to stop the progressive nature of stress-related disease *if they choose to.*

It's easy to picture the development of stress-related illness as a dramatic production. That does not mean that the illness is an act or a fake. Instead, when a sick person's life is viewed over a 2- or 3-year period, it often becomes obvious that the illness has been a long time in coming. There have been signs of trouble for quite some time, and the illness is not a chance occurrence; it has been earned. It's almost as if illness unfolds like the plot of a dramatic production.

We can use the analogy of a three-act play to describe the development of stress-related illness. The illness, as it grows and becomes more serious, looks like a wedge that starts small and gets bigger and bigger. The growth of this illness over time can be divided into three acts (see Figure 3.1).

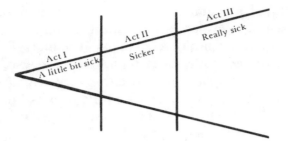

**Figure 3.1    The Three Acts of Illness**

We label what goes on in Act I, "A Little Bit Sick." The name for Act II is "Sicker," and the title for Act III is "Really Sick." Let's take a composite person named "Joe" and follow him through the stages.

*Act I: "A Little Bit Sick"*

Before Act I, Joe is cruising along through life, working hard, attending daily to the stream of obligations and joys with which he has surrounded himself, until he becomes aware of a nagging sense that everything is not right. He is the first person to notice it. He suddenly realizes that he doesn't feel so well. He feels tense, has headaches, has added a few extra pounds, is sleeping restlessly, and feels a sore throat coming on. He is now "a little bit sick."

Then he begins to try to figure out what is going on in his life. He acts as his own doctor, listens to the symptoms, and makes a diagnosis. He may decide that the cause of his problem is that he has been burning the candle at both ends and not getting enough sleep. His fatigue and headaches are the first signs that he's noticed that he's not getting away with this pace unscathed. So he decides on a treatment. "Every night for the next 5 nights, I'm going to bed at 10 o'clock. Then I'll see what happens." He treats himself. If his diagnosis is accurate, based on his knowledge of himself, and if he does follow his treatment plan, then he will probably get well again.

Most of us do this all the time. We go in and out of Act I continually, constantly adjusting our schedule, pace, and ways of taking care of ourselves in light of the feedback our own systems provide. We figure out some home remedies, adjust our schedule, or purchase some of the billions of dollars worth of self-medication sold over the counter (aspirin, Ny-Quil, Tums, Sominex, Kaopectate, heating pads, etc.). Mostly, we get well again.

But let's say that Joe doesn't listen to himself and his body's feedback, and he just keeps pressing on and working too hard. He may get sicker. The next people who begin to notice that something's wrong are his family. One of them says, "Hey, Dad, is something wrong? You don't look well, and you've sure been a grouch." And he replies, "No, nothing's wrong. I am not irritable. I AM NOT IRRITABLE!!" If he listens to the feedback of his family acting as his doctor, he may decide to change his pace and get himself well again.

But if he doesn't attend to his symptoms, he gets sicker, and closer to the end of Act I, and his friends begin to notice. Some friend finally says, "Hey, Joe, when did you last have a checkup?" And he says, "Why?" "Well, you look awful." When people on the outside notice, it begins to get to Joe, so he takes them seriously. His friends act as the doctor. If he follows their advice, he gets well again.

All of us go in and out of Act I over and over again. In Act I people don't define themselves as "sick" and wouldn't bother the doctor. Probably about 60% of the sick people at any given moment are in this stage of illness, or are "just a little bit sick."

Generally, there are few, if any, physicians who spend their time with patients who are a little bit sick. Normally, the only physicians in Act I are the public health doctors, and they are a very small percentage of the total medical personnel in the country. Perhaps the local pharmacist is the major health care provider in this stage. Essentially, the health resources available in Act I are diagnoses and treatments worked out by self, family, and friends (Figure 3.2).

*Act II: "Sicker"*

Let's imagine that Joe does not listen to himself, his family, or his friends. He discovers that he is in the second act of illness when he suddenly says to himself, "I'm sick." He comes to the realization that he needs to do something about it right now. He feels sick. So he decides to call his family physician and see him as soon as possible. If Joe can get an appointment, he sees his physician the same afternoon.

  Let's say his physician is particularly sensitive and he listens to Joe's description of the way his symptoms have been building up over the past months. (This occurrence will be more or less likely, depending on whether his physician takes any time with Joe beyond listening to the list of symptoms and prescribing some medication. In Joe's case it is important that the physician listen, however, because a sensitive and knowledgeable response to Joe's problem will not be possible unless the physician really listens to Joe first.) The physician examines Joe and, when they sit down to talk, he says, "You know, Joe, I really think your fatigue and headaches are related to the stress you're under. Now what can we do to help you make some changes in the way you're living?"

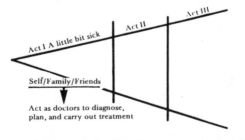

**Figure 3.2   The Resources in Act I**

If Joe listens to him, and the two of them decide on ways to lessen the strain on him, then he probably moves back out of Act II, through Act I, and gets well again.

If the treatment he and his doctor decide on doesn't work, or if he doesn't follow the advice, he may go back three or four times for the same problem. Finally, the physician may say, "Well, Joe, I think you'd better come into the hospital for a workup." So Joe goes into the community hospital for a workup, which may include X rays, extensive laboratory work, perhaps even exploratory surgery. Then another diagnosis and treatment plan are made and, hopefully, Joe gets well again.

Many people go through a large portion of life seldom getting sicker than this. Thus, the family physician can take care of almost all health problems people experience throughout life.

The average person only gets sicker than this once or twice in his/her life. The family doctor and the community hospital are able to take care of most people's medical needs.

Probably about 30% of the sick people in our country at any given moment are in the second stage of illness. In this second act, the major health resources available are the family physician, prescription medications, and the community hospital (Figure 3.3).

*Act III: "Really Sick"*

A small percentage of people get sicker than Act II and move into Act III. Let's say that happened to Joe. The family physician finally doesn't know what to try next. He feels that he can't handle the problem any longer, and he says, "Joe, I would like for you to see a friend of mine who is a specialist." Now Joe is in Act III, which is the domain of the specialist and the teaching and research hospital.

Joe sees the specialist. The specialist focuses on the

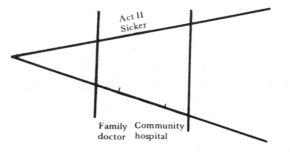

**Figure 3.3   The Resources in Act II**

problem; by now Joe's problem is pretty big, so it is obvious. We must be careful not to be critical of the family
doctor who couldn't define the problem fully, since he saw
Joe when it was much smaller. The specialist is able to
recognize and deal with Joe's problem because it's big now,
and because the specialist knows this particular type of
problem very well.

Occasionally, if Joe is really a rare case, the specialist
can't handle it alone, and after dealing with it awhile says,
"You know, I think you'd better come to the research hospital." So Joe would go to the research and teaching hospital, which is often connected with a medical school, or at
least a residency program, and there he would see not just
specialists, but the superspecialists, or the subspecialists.
Joe probably won't understand much of what they talk
about. But he shouldn't worry; most superspecialists are so
engrossed in one aspect of one type of disease that they
don't understand each other very well.

Anyway, the specialists and subspecialists on Joe's
"case" would put their collective heads together and do
some remarkable work with his disease and then send him
back to his family doctor, and then to his friends and family,
and he finally gets well again.

Probably only about 10% of the sick population at any
given moment is sick enough to need the care of specialists,
subspecialists, and the technology of a teaching and research hospital (Figure 3.4).

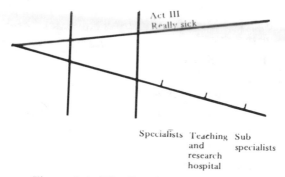

**Figure 3.4    The Resources in Act III**

At the far end of Act III looms Act IV, "The Final Curtain." It is the realm of undertakers and ministers. Most of us spend our lives trying to stay out of this Act.

## The Distribution of Sickness and the Distribution of Services

The problem with the present system of allocating health care resources becomes immediately evident when a wedge depicting the distribution of health care resources is super-imposed on a wedge depicting the distribution of all sick people (Figure 3.5).

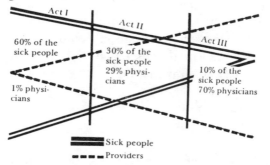

**Figure 3.5    The Distribution of Sickness and of Services**

The heavy lined wedge stands for all the people in America who are ill at any given moment. There are the sick people, starting with those who are a little bit sick, then those who are sicker and, finally, the really sick. Approximately 60% of the sick people in America in any one day are in Act I. They are doing all kinds of things to take care of themselves, such as home remedies, sleep, exercise, and the rest. In Act I, however, we have approximately 1% of the doctors—those in epidemiology and preventive medicine (dotted line wedge).

When we move to Act II, we find roughly 30% of the sick people and approximately the same percentage of doctors; we'll make it 29%. These are generalists, family practice physicians, internists, pediatricians, and so forth.

Finally, in Act III there are only 10% of the sick people, but approximately 70% of the doctors.

These observations are borne out by health statistics. A 1960 survey found that out of 1000 people during any given month, 750 will have one minor illness, 250 will consult a physician, nine will be admitted to a hospital, five will be referred to another physician, and one will be admitted to a university medical center. This study concluded that 25% of the population has apparent need for some medical care each month. Only 1.5% need hospital admission or specialist care.

Therefore, 98% of the population, during a month, either has no need for professional health care or has need only for services of a primary health care nature (Andreopoulos, 1974). This primary care service needs drastic expansion.

## The Call for Change

The priorities on which the allocation of health care resources is based need to be revised. The allocation of resources needs to be reversed. Much more attention must be placed both on concentrating medical resources in Acts I and II and on utilizing the unused auxiliary health care and helping resources that already exist in Acts I and II.

*THE TREND TOWARD CHANGE—MOVEMENT TOWARD EARLIER STAGES.*
For years, based partly on the prestige and glamor of speciality work and partly on the money available for work in Act III, the distribution of health care resources has been increasingly focused on Act III, the subspecialists and the teaching and research hospitals. Fortunately, today, due to a number of factors—not the least of which is consumer dissatisfaction—a heartening trend toward movement of medical resources into the earlier acts of illness is evident.

Many physicians are seeing the need to become involved in earlier stages of illness and prevention instead of focusing on cure after the fact. Specialists have tended not to see people until the third act of illness. It's like going to a theater and getting there at 10 P.M. when Acts I and II are over and they're just starting Act III, and so they sit back in their seats and think to themselves, "What could have happened in Acts I and II to make them say what they're saying now in Act III?" That's essentially what the specialist is up against. Many specialists would love to see people earlier, in Act II instead of Act III.

Many general family practice physicians are talking more of prevention today. They would love to be in Act I instead of Act II. For years, not only have there been very few physicians interested in Act I, but most physicians have scoffed at their colleagues practicing in Act I, in the area of preventive medicine. Courses in preventive medicine have scarcely caught the imagination of most medical students. They have been full of epidemiology and health statistics —not very exciting. There has never been the glamor in teaching people proper nutrition as there has been in open heart surgery. Yet there's a great deal of wisdom in the adage, "An ounce of prevention is worth a pound of cure."

The revolution that's beginning to take place in medicine is characterized by a renewed interest in prevention and a desire to move back into earlier stages of illness.

*THE REVOLUTION IN MEDICAL EDUCATION.*    Way out at the farthest end of Act III, where the subspecialists do their work on rare diseases and spectacular treatments—where less than a tenth of 1% of the sick population is—that is where the teaching and research hospitals function. That's where the medical schools are located. That's where we teach young people to become doctors. These students are taught almost entirely by superspecialists, whose interests lie primarily in only a small subpart of their speciality. As a result, the medical student in the past rarely worked with general practitioners. In fact, G.P.s were looked on as inferiors, with no special expertise to offer. Medical students were taught by scientific researchers from each of the 20–30 small speciality areas. No one helped students to see the broad perspective of the whole person. Is it any wonder that young doctors at times tend to view people merely as physiological systems and functions?

At present, this trend is beginning to show signs of change. A whole new speciality, the family practice speciality, has arisen within the past 10 years. Over half of the medical schools in the country have instituted family practice residency programs within the past 6 years.

The trend of the past has been to overtrain medical students in urban teaching and research hospitals, where they see only critically ill people and where they're surrounded by superspecialists doing research. Today medical educators are trying to move the training out into the community hospitals where physicians in training meet sick people with "ordinary problems." These students and residents are meeting family physicians and are learning to see and treat whole families as units. In Chicago there are now six community hospitals that take medical students on a rotating basis. The physician graduating in the future will be better acquainted with and better equipped to deal with the myriad of psychological, environmental, and stress-related forms of diseases that are manifested in the early stages of illness.

*THE NEED TO UTILIZE AUXILIARY RESOURCES ALREADY ACTIVE IN ACT I.*   The movement toward focusing medical practice and medical teaching in Act II is necessary. But what about Act I? Who will be available to offer care to people who are only "a little bit sick?" Do we need more and more physicians who focus on Act I?

No! Sending physicians who have 6–10 years of technical training in sickness care into Act I would be foolish. There are, however, already many people in addition to friends and family who are interested in health care at the Act I level: public health nurses, counselors, teachers, and clergy. These professional groups focus on health care instead of sickness care. For the most part, these people have not been considered seriously as part of the health care system.

Utilization and coordination of efforts with persons in the nonmedical health care professions will bring the proportion of providers in Act I more in line with the proportion of sick people who are in the first act of illness (see Figure 3.6). This utilization of the nonmedical providers will also offer renewed attention to social, emotional, and spiritual factors that are so central in the development of life-style and stress-related disease.

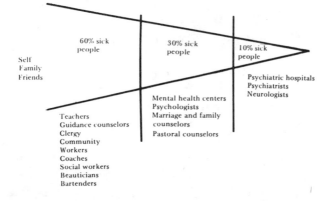

**Figure 3.6   The Distribution of Nonmedical Health Care Resources**

The clergy and the local schoolteachers as well as many others get to know whole families, and they maintain the relationship over a period of time. They know the stresses and strains people are under. They know when grandpa died, when the youngest child left home, when all three toddlers have had the flu, when dad lost his job. These professional people are in touch with the stresses of life pressing on people that contribute greatly to the onset of illness in its earliest stages. Their knowledge and history with people must be tapped and taken seriously in the health care system.

Generally, physicians have known very little, and cared less, about how to utilize resources of professions other than their own. I have yet to hear a physician react with anything but surprise when I ask whether he/she had ever thought of involving the family's minister in treatment. But involve him/her we must. It is not necessary for a huge percentage of physicians to suddenly start working in Act I of illness. This involvement would not efficiently utilize the high-level technical training of physicians. It is necessary, however, to take seriously the educators, clergy, counselors, nurse practitioners, and others with expertise and interest in the preventive efforts so essential for assisting persons in the first act of illness. These "auxiliary" health care providers can assist persons in managing their stress and in changing their life-styles—before they get sicker.

*REISSUING THE CALL FOR CHANGE IN PRIORITIES.*    The health care system (presently a sickness care system), which in the recent past has been focused primarily on Act III, needs to change. Much more attention must be given by the medical community, public funding agencies, and private foundations to establishing priorities in Acts I and II. The technology of medicine has now been developed to the point where we can keep people alive for months just by machines. Now is the time to turn attention and full energy to changing the feudal-style delivery system and developing it to a high level of efficiency that matches the technology. For the technology to begin to make a major impact on the general health level and quality of life of the U.S. population, the delivery system must be perfected.

The revolution of health care will involve a shift of priorities from the sickness to the health end of the spectrum.

In this process the churches, schools, and community agencies can play a big part. Out where people work, live, and play, we have to find ways to make a teamwork approach to *health* care acceptable and easily available to the public. We must pay increased attention to the life-style pressures and the signs of disease exhibited in the non-physical aspects of living: emotions, social relationships, faith, and the like. Attention to the management of stress in the early stages of sickness will help people to interrupt the progressive development of disease and make it unnecessary for them to move into the second and third acts of illness before they get help.

## SUMMARY

There are positive forces pushing for a revolution and a return to primary medicine. Consumers are outraged. State legislators are beginning to revolt and vote money for the development of primary care physicians within their states. Medical students are demanding more courses in family medicine, counseling, and psychogenetic illness.

There are changes brewing. Still, for the most part at this point in history, the medical system is of little help for your health until you're quite sick. Without question, the system is a partial cause of the trouble.

How did we get here? Where does the fault lie? It could be placed with the medical establishment. It could be placed with the consumer. It could even be placed with churches and clergy, educational institutions and their teachers, or governmental agencies and administrators for their failure to risk involvement and investment for change. But what's the purpose of placing the blame? The proper question is not "Who's at fault?", but "Where do we go from here? What can be done now?"

It is important to acknowledge that there are presently some real and serious problems in the delivery of medical care services. There are some factors that cry out for change. Health care providers are not entirely happy with the present situation. Patients (the consumers) certainly aren't satisfied. There is a problem. There must be better ways to deliver health care. They must be found.

If we are to develop a higher-quality health care in our country that is characterized by easy availability, personalized human concern, and the whole person focus, the system will have to change. Whether the result should be neighborhood outpatient clinics as satellites of hospitals, new types of nonphysician primary care practitioners, a new type of physician, or an entirely new system, we do not know. If the problems of the present system, which cause anger and frustration for both providers and patients and thus at times decrease instead of increase health, are to be dealt with constructively, then the demands of the consumer for a more readily available, more personalized, and more wholistic approach to health needs must begin to receive primary attention in the earlier stages of illness.

Without question, the system for making the health care resources of our country available to people when and where they need them is out of balance and very inefficient, and is the cause of some of the trouble. But such a system would never have been developed if it didn't fit the American priorities—priorities that overemphasize technical miracles and dramatic response to critical emergencies and underemphasize the "more mundane" focus on health education, prevention, early examination, and the individual patient's responsibility for living a health-producing life-style.

The dramatic has gotten a disproportionate share of the health care dollar, because the American people would rather not think about their health until they are really sick. Then any money expenditure is acceptable to cure them.

The problem is not only the system. The problems of the system are based on a mechanical, physiological concept of health and illness that does not take seriously the role of stress and life-style in the onset of disease; that does not place emphasis on the individual's responsibility for maintaining health. If we are to return an appropriate focus of the health care effort to the earlier stages of illness, the definitions of health and illness on which our present priorities are based will have to change. If we are to get to the heart of the trouble with health care today, we will have to move beyond criticizing the system and making it the scapegoat.

We will have to search out some new understandings of, definitions for, and approaches to the meaning of health and illness. We will need to develop concepts for health care that take seriously the whole person and the dynamic relationships among stress, life-style, and disease.

## Chapter 4

# OUR CONCEPTS OF HEALTH
# AND ILLNESS ARE OUTDATED

What is really behind all the gripes of consumers and providers, behind all the inadequacies of the delivery system? Is there an error, common to and cause of all of these symptoms?

Perhaps all the efforts of our modern health care, magnificent as they are, are based on a faulty, limited definition of people, of life, health, and illness. Our challenge, if we are ever going to change the system and respond more adequately to the needs of providers and patients—needs that are expressed in the form of complaints—is to look for a more humanistic view of health, illness, the healing process, and the role of health providers; this view must take the whole person seriously as an integrated human being.

The efforts to solve the health care problems have been enormous. They have also been well intentioned. But they have been misplaced. We haven't solved the troubles of the health care system in the past 10 years, but it isn't because we haven't tried.

## THE PROBLEM OF MINDSET

Why haven't our efforts produced a better form of health care? Why hasn't this radical, unprecedented expenditure of resources resulted in a higher level of health?

In order to look for a possible answer, I'd like to use an analogy from counseling practice. A hunch for an area in which reasons for our present dilemma in health care may be found lies in knowledge of the ways individuals go about solving their emotional, life-style problems.

Clients come to a therapist, counselor, pastor, physician, *not* because they are lazy and haven't tried to solve their own problems; instead, they come to someone else for help *after* they have tried everything they can think of and nothing has helped. They come because they don't know what to try next.

The problem is they have been working out of a specific limited mindset. An analysis of the attempts they have made will often show a pattern. Usually people consider few alternatives. They center on one or two ways of problem solving that fit with their habitual way of viewing problems, and they keep on trying variations of the same until they run out of patience. The job of the counselor, therapist, pastor, physician, is to help them redefine the situation so that new alternatives for action, for correction of the problem, may be found.

Is it possible that we Americans have been searching for solutions to the problems of health care only within a small segment of the possible alternatives? Is it possible that the health care system is the result of a limited, faulty mindset about human health and illness? Is it possible that breaking this mindset could help us to find new, more successful approaches to promoting health?

In order to examine these questions, let's look at another analogy—this time in the creative problem-solving methodology developed in industry and marketing programs. Creative problem solving begins with exercises to stimulate ways of redefining the problem before looking for a solution. When the problem is redefined, new solutions may be immediately evident. Ways are needed to break the mindset toward the problem that has developed in previous attempts at solution finding. The goal is to alter the habit patterns that have governed all courses of actions attempted—actions that have produced no results.

Let's take an example. A company making can openers has a problem. They are not selling enough can openers. The designers come together to plan a better can opener. First they plan a ball-bearing one, then a permanently lubricated one, then a pearl-handled one, then a mink-covered one and, finally, an electric one. Their hope, of course, is that they can make a can opener which will corner the limited can opening market and sell more products.

But they have only limited success, until one day someone redefines the problem. "Our goal is not to sell can openers. Our goal is to make a profit in opening cans." The flip-top tab can is born, can openers become obsolete, and the company has a corner on the market.

Can we who are concerned about the ills and shortcomings of our present health care system learn from the approach of creative problem solving? We have little to lose. More of the same, it seems, will not help.

Can we who watch the pain and disease in the lives of those we attempt to help, we who see how limited is our ability to bring health and quality of life to others under our present mindset (our present health care system), can we afford not to look for a better way?

Can we attempt to redefine the problem in the present health care system and investigate the complaints that indicate needs that are not being met?

Can we redefine the problems, hear the complaints of patients, physicians, clergy, therapists, educators, hear the needs underneath the complaints, and redefine the problem in such a way as to find a creative solution or set of solutions, or at least a direction for our search in which a solution may be found?

Can we somehow break through our mindset in thinking about health and illness, in thinking about health care, doctors, clinics, hospitals, and medications, so that some solutions that will really improve the health of Americans can be found?

We might as well try. Building bigger hospitals and training more physicians, who go to school longer and learn more and more about less and less, hasn't cured our ills. More and more energy expended in the same old patterns hasn't helped. More and more efficient technology hasn't given us the quality of life and health that we seek. All of the enormous system has become, by the weight of its efforts, the generator and perpetrator of additional problems, additional causes of disease. We might as well try something new.

## THE CHALLENGE TO REDEFINE CONCEPTS

It seems likely that a redefinition of the problem will require us to examine our accepted cultural definition of health and health care.

Very possibly all of the efforts of our billions of dollars and millions of health care providers to create better health are based on a faulty definition of health and illness. Our efforts are based on a very limited view of what makes people sick and what makes a life healthy and worth living.

I submit that the reason we as a culture are in poor health, that the reason our enormous attacks on the ills of our people have not worked so far, is that we have based our efforts on a mindset of technology alone. With the great advance in technology, we seem to have become hypnotized by all that technology can do. We seem to have lost our judgment, our ability to make rational choices in the use of technology. It controls us and makes decisions for people, instead of people being in control and making the decisions.

We have, as a culture, grown to have more faith in computer printouts than in people. We trust the accuracy of machines more than persons. If you don't believe it, just try to get a correction made on a bank statement or on a charge account.

In health care, too, we have developed a pervasive attitude that human bodies are like machines, that when the trouble with the machine is found to be a worn or ill-functioning part, it can be replaced and proper functioning will be restored.

As a culture we act out three unsupportable assumptions about health care: we define *human health* as having to do only with the body and its functions; we define *human illness* as produced by malfunctioning physical components; we define *health care* as focused on chemically restoring homeostatic physical balance, excising and replacing broken parts.

I believe that these definitions are faulty, hopelessly incomplete, and unable to explain health or illness or the activities of meaningful human life, and are the basis of the problem in health care today.


## TENTATIVE STEPS TOWARD A NEW MINDSET

I suspect, based on the tenets of technology, that we will never find solutions to the problems of the health care system and will never really significantly and lastingly affect the general level of health experienced within our society until we redefine the problem. We will find some solutions to the problem by redefining our assumptions about the nature of people, and by finding the contributors to, and effects of, both health and illness; not within the context of the dissection of people into microscopic components, but within a perspective of health and illness as related to the whole, interrelated human person, interacting with other persons and the environment.

We will not obtain better health or quality health care until we redefine our view of health and illness to include all aspects of personhood, in addition to the physical, feelings, beliefs, friendships, environment, ideas, goals, disappointments, dreams, fears, values, choices, and the like. These must be included in the definition of health and illness.

I suggest that when we begin to search for a redefinition of health as wholeness and illness as brokenness, then we (all of us from a variety of disciplines) will be able to see possibilities for new alternatives and potential for new solutions to the problems of health care that have not as yet occurred to any of us.

By following this path of redefinition of health and illness, priorities may be reversed. We may, for instance, choose to spend $100 on health planning before people get sick instead of $3,000 on surgery to repair the damage of the sickness. New cooperation between professions will emerge with new definitions of the scope of health care. Perhaps new styles of cooperative, coordinated care will result when health care providers broaden their perspective of the factors contributing to health.

I suggest that the assumptions underlying a wholistic approach to health will lead us to expenditures, efforts, and treatment plans far different from today's comfortable (but unhealthy), antiproductive patterns.

We will have to join together in a different, perhaps, uncomfortable attempt to construct a view of health, illness, healing, and treatment that, in the breadth of its perspective, encompasses the human spirit as well as the human body. We must establish a definition of health and health care that encompasses the "spirit" dimension of a living, breathing human being as well as physical systems and chemical reactions.

## SOME COMPONENTS IN THE NEW MINDSET

Although it is premature to lay out a well-formulated redefinition of health and illness, there are at least three issues that will certainly become key building blocks in the health care concepts of the future.

*1.   The Health Care of the Future Will Certainly be Based on the Premise That Each Person is Ultimately Responsible For Himself/Herself and For His/Her Measure of Health.*

In traditional medicine patients and physicians make a sordid kind of deal with each other. The patient promises to abide by whatever the doctor says, without questioning, without understanding what is wrong, in exchange for the subtle promise by the physician that he/she will heal the problem without effort or pain for the patient. The physician is caught in the act of saying "Here, here now, don't you worry, this pill will take care of everything." Counselors, pastors, nurses, and social workers are often caught in the same "game."

Unfortunately, real healing doesn't happen this way. The physician can't deliver on that promise, and the patient is robbed of the opportunity or heavy responsibility (whichever you choose to make it) of understanding the meaning of his/her own illness and making appropriate life-style decisions in the face of it. When people get angry about the sordid deal they made, they sue.

The authoritarian, parental model is beginning to break down. That which is truly revolutionary and basic in the new health care will have at its center the tenet that the patient is responsible for his/her sickness and healing. The physician is the coach.

The shift in research emphasis today away from focusing on the "bug" that attacks people and makes them sick exemplifies this change. The most recent research trend is to study the host, the person, who makes a receptive home for the disease. Why do some catch the "bug" while others do not?

The emphasis on patient responsibility is also evident in the infrequent, but growing, number of medical and counseling centers where the patient's ideas are considered seriously and where the information on the charts belongs to the patient, not the medical system and the medical provider.

Along with this emphasis will come a new form of diagnostic questioning. No longer will the questions be directed only by the provider on specific facts: "How long have you had it?" "When does it hurt?" "Did your parents have it?" "Have you done anything about it?"

The new diagnostic questions will take seriously the knowledge and the responsibility which the patient has for his/her own illness: "What do you think is wrong with you?" "Why did you get this disease?" "Why did you get this disease now?" "What does it mean in your life?" "What would it cost you to give up this ailment?"

These questions affirm that the patient didn't "pick up" the disease, but earned or chose it. This kind of questioning will be difficult for both providers and patients to learn, but it will be a necessary skill in helping people to take responsibility for themselves.

*2.    The Health Care of The Future Will Certainly Be Based On The Premise That Illness and Health Is A Function Of Every Aspect Of Life, Not Just The Physical.*

For the past years medicine, for all practical purposes, has been considered to be all there is to the health care field. The growing data on life-style and the influence of stress factors on dis-ease within every aspect of life returns physical medicine to a limited place as only one aspect of the health care field.

At this point, medical research itself has shown that life-style habits, stress, hope, will, and meaningful close relationships all significantly affect the individual's susceptivity to disease and response-ability to be healed. However, little has been done in the traditional medical practice to take these data seriously or to include attention to these factors in the treatment plans that are implemented.

Medicine of the future will not look only for a one-to-one correspondence between an individual and a disease, will not separate body, mind, and spirit, will not only find broken parts and mend them, and will not be an isolated approach. Medicine of the future will treat the person in context—in the context of environment and social and cultural atmosphere. It will take the will and the belief system seriously.

No longer will "asthmatic," "gastric colitis," "hypertensive," or (heaven forbid) the epidemic nondisease "hypoglycemia" be enough of a diagnosis to specify appropriate treatment. The medicine of the future will add a new set of diagnostic terms—words that describe the human spirit and will include "loneliness," "guilty," "uncommited," "powerless," and the like alongside the traditional terminology.

No longer will treatment center on Digitalis, Valium, X ray, and so on. Treatment will be supplemented with making friends, giving of one's self in love, hobbies, meditation, and worship.

The spiritual side of life will again be seen as the organizing principle, and providers will ask appropriate questions.

What is important to you? (Values)

What do you believe? (Faith)

What are you willing to expend yourself on? (Commitment)

What are you willing to give up? (Surrender)

These questions will again be central to the meaning of health and life and will be utilized for the promotion of health and stimulation to increase the quality of life.

The health care of the future will make diagnostic judgments and interventions within every aspect of life, not just the physical. Health will be seen as a measure of the total life—the total person.

*3.   The Health Care of the Future Will Certainly Be Based On A New, Updated Understanding Of The Relationship Between The Physical, The Mental, and The Spiritual As Merely Different Forms of Life Energy.*

Presently, the health care model looks at the physical body entirely as a material entity, something that can be weighed, measured, cut open, and manipulated. It is governed by the "laws of nature." This limited understanding of the material is akin to the assumptions of Newtonian physics. Matter is matter, and there isn't much more to say about it. Just work with it long enough and find out the properties of each element.

Well, Newtonian physics is fairly outmoded. Einstein changed the course of physics. We now know (and have known for 30 years) that matter, light, mind, heat and electricity are all merely different forms of the same thing— energy. Our medicine is presently based on a concept that is 30 years outdated.

When we begin to get a sense of the truth that our body is only one form of our energy, it isn't so difficult to imagine how the mind affects the body; how will power can change the course of an illness; how some people can, and have, healed cancer by visualizing the healing process within themselves; how meditation, relaxation, and prayer can change physical health; and how ancient Eastern energy-flow theory may be true.

When we begin to accept that our body is only one form of our energy, then it isn't hard to begin to see that health is more than that which we can see and measure. It's a spirit quality, an energy flow, not just bodily functions.

If our health relates to energy, then it's not hard to see that just as an electric wire needs contact in order for electricity to flow through it, so also do people need people. People need contact, care, and love in order to be healthy. People need to let energy flow from themselves to others in order to be energized themselves. When there's no contact and no exchange of energy and love, can symptoms of tiredness, depression, and ill-health be far behind?

When we begin to understand that our body is only one form of our energy, then it isn't so antiscientific to begin to consider the influx of the spirit, the miraculous healings, and the resurrection of the dead promised in the Judeo-Christian scriptures.

When we begin to feel that our body is only one form of energy, then we see that nothing is against the laws of nature—only against our understanding of those laws.

The health care of the future will certainly be based on a new updated respect for energy as the organic unity between the physical, the mental, and the spiritual. Health care in the future will confirm a belief in the power of the individual will and the healing effects of care and love exchanged between people.

## THE VISION

How can we begin to solve some of the problems of the health care system? It's going to take a revision in our thinking. It's going to take a redefinition of the concepts of health and and illness.

I suspect that we will begin to find some full measure of health again:

when breathing is not only inhaling and exhaling, → but a way of expressing "I am . . . (inhale) love"(exhale) when breathing is a mystery of God, the infusion of God's spirit

when hearts are not only highly elastic, supremely efficient pumps for blood, → but symbols of love, hope, joy, and grief

when feet, hands, arms, and legs, are not only appendages to be reset by an orthopod, → but are parts of ourselves that assist in the translation of goals, values, and priorities into constructive action and love

when our eyes, ears, mouth, skin, and tongue are not only mechanical organs of sense, → but are our windows for participation with each other in the mystery of life and the enjoyment of contact and the exchange of love

when death is not only expiration (the cessation of breathing, heartbeats, brain-wave activity, or whatever the current mechanical definition of death happens to be), → but when death is the transformation of a self into a beyond of the universe—a return unto God

when behavior is not a consequence of prior conditioning in the evolutionary process, → but a choice, from the crucible of our values, for which we are responsible

I believe that we will begin to find some solutions to the problems of our health care system:

when a person is no longer an assemblage of parts that can be fully discovered through minute scrutiny—piece by piece

→ but when a person is again seen as a whole to be loved and contacted with awe

## SUMMARY

Who is going to supply this new (but very old), radical (but simple), more adequate, more fully human definition of health? Who is going to supply the proper questions, the wholistic terminology, the ways for helping people to be responsible for themselves, for helping them to return to commitments beyond themselves to find meaning in life— and ultimate health? Who is going to help them to learn to love one another and to heal each other's brokenness?

I believe that it's time that we in the medical and auxiliary health professions start solving the needs of modern medicine by returning to some sense, by forcing the recognition of the human spirit dimension in every aspect of health and disease that is manifested in our society, individual and corporate, and by making our healing presence felt in every aspect of care for every manifestation of disease.

Where do we go from here? Is this kind of reasoning —that it's not the complaints of providers and patients, not the shortcomings of the system that is really the root of the trouble in the health care system—sensible? Is it possible that a wholistic mindset is needed before much progress will be made toward finding solutions to the problems of modern health care? I think the answer is, "Yes."

Is this kind of thinking utopian? I think the answer is, "No." New concepts are being discussed. Alternate, more wholistic models for the delivery of health care consistent with these new concepts have already been developed.

The next several chapters describe one of these alternate models, the Wholistic Health Center project. The Wholistic Health Center is a successful experiment in applying the principles of wholistic health in a primary care setting. It gets beyond the limited mindset of technology and explores new concepts and tests new care methodologies. It's an innovation, yet it remains part of the medical care system. It responds to the primary complaints of both patients and providers. It's an experimental demonstration that works.

But there are other possibilities for the return to and application of whole-person health care principles. This is just a beginning. The surface has hardly been touched. Other possibilities exist for those who will seek them.

## Chapter 5

# THE WHOLISTIC HEALTH CENTER: AN ALTERNATE HEALTH CARE MODEL

## THE NEW MINDSET IN ACTION

New methodologies for utilizing the diagnosis of the problems as well as the concepts and principles of whole-person health care must be developed and tested in action-research models.

Instead of calling for revolution, crying out for the overthrow of the medical system as it exists today, and replacing it with cultic, extreme, nontechnical forms of healing, it seems prudent to search for ways in which the present system for delivering care can be adapted to include a renewed focus on the wholeness of the disease and health process, a focus on the whole person.

One such alternative model for the delivery of whole-person health is the Wholistic Health Center, a model that intentionally fits itself into the context of the medical care system.

The Wholistic Health Centers are church-based, family practice medical care facilities that utilize an interdisciplinary team of physicians, pastoral counselors, and nurses who focus on all aspects of an individual's health needs.

Wholistic health care as practiced in the Centers is based on the metaphysical affirmation of body, mind, and spirit integrated in a whole that is independent of and greater than the sum of its parts. In practice, wholistic health care means actively searching with a patient all dimensions of his/her life (physical, emotional, intellectual, spiritual, interpersonal) for causes and symptoms of disease, then creatively exploring these same modalities for treatment strategies to restore or maintain health.

## AN OVERVIEW

Presently there are four model "test" Centers in the United States: Springfield, Ohio (started in 1970), Hinsdale, Illinois (1973), Woodridge, Illinois (1974), and Mendota, Illinois (1976). Four more sites are in the process of development and will open during 1977–1978.

The Centers were funded originally through private grant monies. Since 1973, they have been sponsored by the University of Illinois at the Medical Center, Chicago, and have received start-up support from the W. K. Kellogg Foundation. The Centers in the western suburbs of Chicago, Hinsdale and Woodridge, are self-supporting. Each Center is intended to reach the self-support level within 12-24 months.

Emphasizing health education, early examination, and prevention, and specializing in the treatment and care of the whole person, the Wholistic Health Center project is intended to be a limited but creative attempt to respond to some of the weaknesses in the present system of delivering health care. It is an effort to take seriously the influence of mind and spirit on physical health and, by utilizing the concepts of wholistic care and family medicine, to develop innovative methods for delivering personal health care. The project is in search of methods for providing higher-quality, more complete primary health care in earlier stages of illness to larger numbers of individuals at less cost.

## Comparison with Other Medical Facilities

The Wholistic Health Center project is a venture that is, on the one hand, regular and commonplace and, on the other, an experiment that is unique and exciting. The effort consists of traditional models of medical and counseling care combined in a very nontraditional manner and setting, based on sound philosophical principles. This results in an experience for patients that is both similar to other health care experiences and, at the same time unique and totally different in focus.

The Wholistic Health Center is, simply, a family practice medical clinic. The physicians who presently practice within the Centers practice just as any other physicians. They see people for medical problems, keep records, recommend and interpret laboratory tests, prescribe medications, consult with specialists, hospitalize patients, make hospital rounds, and respond to an endless round of phone questions. They consider themselves family (general) doctors for our patients. Their practice involves the same activities and procedures, demands the same interests and skills, and creates the same problems as most any other general medical practice.

However, instead of locating their offices near their homes or in large medical clinic buildings, our physicians have located their offices in church buildings. The examining rooms are the same 10 X 10 foot cubicles lined with diagnostic equipment and instruments that are found in any physician's office. The consulting rooms, waiting rooms, and office space all appear similar to any other physician's office. However, special attention is given to furnishing rooms to encourage in-depth discussion instead of hurried efficiency. All rooms except the two examining rooms are utilized in the evenings by health education classes and on Sunday mornings by church education classes.

The pastoral counselors, nurses, and secretary/receptionists carry out many of the same professional and administrative tasks as their counterparts in any medical office or mental health agency.

Fees for services are similar to those charged by other health care professionals in the area. The four full-time salaried staff members (physician, nurse, pastoral counselor, and secretary) are augmented by other professional volunteers who serve 1/2 day or 1 day per week. Following the initial expenditure of $5000-$7000 for equipment and remodeling, each individual clinic operates on an annual budget of approximately $85,000.

On the one hand, the Wholistic Health Center is not very different from other medical or counseling offices. On the other hand, however, the staff has put a lot of time, effort, and emotion into making the Wholistic Health Centers very different from other medical and/or counseling offices that we have known.

Is the difference our interest in the whole person? Is it our teamwork approach? Is it our attempt to focus on health and not on illness? Is it our taking the patient seriously as an adult? Perhaps all of these plus other factors, contribute. The uniqueness lies mainly in the conscious attempt, which is regularly reexamined, to take our name, *Wholistic* Health Center, seriously. The focus is on the whole person (or family) not just a piece. It is on health, not on illness and disease. It is a Center designed to coordinate services for all health care needs.

Central to the treatment of any disease within the Center is the teamwork approach. The patient, the nurse, the physician, and the pastoral counselor are each taken seriously as members of the planning and treatment team, and each is expected to bring his/her unique expertise to bear on the problem as needed.

## The Historical Development

It's somewhat difficult to describe the Wholistic Health Center adequately in a few introductory paragraphs. It's probably almost as difficult to read a few paragraphs and develop an instantly clear picture of this experiment in whole-person health care. A short description of the historical development should help to set the context (Tubesing, 1976).

THE INITIAL PILOT CLINIC.    In response to the growing inadequacy of medical care delivery, especially for inner-city residents, the pilot "church clinic" was established in a high unemployment, disadvantaged area of Springfield, Ohio in 1970. A volunteer staff of doctors, nurses, and clergy-counselors was recruited and began providing free primary medical care in basement Sunday school rooms, two of which had been equipped as makeshift examining rooms.

The approach to patient health needs was wholistic. Through the integration of pastoral counseling with medical care, illness was treated in its relationship to the whole person and in the context of the social, emotional, and spiritual stresses experienced by the patients. After 6 months, services were expanded to include an eye and dental clinic as well as legal aid.

Within 3 months, the clinic was crowded with patients on its one afternoon opening per week. By the second year, hours were expanded to 4-½ days each week. Presently, the Springfield clinic still operates at this pace.

Before long the large numbers of patients and the feedback from patient attitude surveys, as well as the decreasing use of the area emergency vehicles, demonstrated the success of the church clinic in this neighborhood. The church clinic was, in fact, responding successfully to a human need by providing low-cost but sound medical care that focused on the whole person (Holinger & Westberg, 1975).

*THE CHALLENGE FOR FURTHER TESTING.*     As nationwide interest in this project grew, it became obvious that churches and synagogues throughout the country could be utilized as clinic sites with the same benefits of decreased capitalization and less regular overhead cost. Such church-based clinics could also enlist volunteers in developing a wholistic, more complete kind of care.

Still to be demonstrated, however, was whether the Springfield clinic was successful merely because it was a free clinic in an area of inadequate medical care, or whether the community response was based also on the qualitative difference (i.e., the added dimensions of whole-person care, listening, and the multiprofessional teamwork approach).

The challenge became clear. If the wholistic type of care practiced in this clinic was to influence primary care medicine, and if it was to be demonstrated that the wholistic approach was an advantageous one, the project would have to be transplanted to a neighborhood where people have a choice about the kind of health care they prefer. Would people both choose and pay for wholistic care offered in a church-based clinic when there were other acceptable alternatives?

*THE EXPANSION.*     In search of an answer to this question, the metropolitan Chicago area was chosen as a target location. Although Dr. Granger Westberg, the prime mover in the project, was well known in Chicago, the search for start-up grant monies, for a supporting grantee institution, and for appropriate suburban church locations took 1 year of full-time effort.

Early in 1973, Dr. Edward Lichter, Chairman of the Department of Preventive Medicine and Community Health, University of Illinois at the Medical Center, Chicago, responded positively to the project and gained the necessary institutional support. In April 1973, the W.K. Kellogg Foundation authorized a $390,000 4-year grant that funded a coordinating office and initial capital for two Wholistic Health Centers in the metropolitan Chicago area.

In choosing a test community for this model, a number of factors were outlined as important. It was felt that the community should (1) be well-doctored, (2) have a good local hospital, (3) be predominantly middle-upper income, and (4) comprise a medically sophisticated population. If a church-based Wholistic Health Center in such an area could support itself within 3 years, the venture would be judged a success on at least one parameter.

Hinsdale, Illinois, a western suburb of Chicago, was chosen as the first site. Within this middle-upper income community are located an extremely high ratio of general practitioners and specialists, as well as an excellent hospital with an educational focus—the Hinsdale Sanitarium and Hospital. The clinic was opened at the Union Church (United Church of Christ) of Hinsdale in September 1973.

Although plans called for opening the second test clinic in a rural area, a truly rural community was not located within a feasible distance from Chicago for adequate development and administration during the early phase. Therefore, Woodridge, a new bedroom suburb characterized by extremely high mobility and lack of medical services, was chosen as the second test site. This clinic opened in September 1974 at the Woodridge United Methodist Church.

A third full-time Center opened in rural Mendota, Illinois in December 1976. All three Wholistic Health Centers presently operate in affiliation with each other and engage in similar styles for delivering whole-person health care. Each, of course, has incorporated unique care programs that have contributed to the overall development of wholistic health care methodology. All are presently full-time, totally self-supporting Centers.

## THE STYLE OF CARE

Probably 50% of the patients who enter a doctor's office for medical care have problems whose causes lie more in the realm of the spirit than the body. Certainly all physical illnesses produce resultant life stress, anxiety, and perhaps emotional or spiritual upheaval. Most life stress problems, if serious enough, eventually affect one's physical health. The stresses and strains of living (working, raising a family, making friends, growing up, growing older, suffering loss, etc.) are powerful factors that influence a person's total health and quality of life. Most people have a sense that spiritual factors (the meaning they find in life, their feelings of love, joy, hope, etc.) profoundly affect not only their outlook on life, but also their physical energy and health.

### The Basic Care Style

The Wholistic Health Center staff attempts to utilize this information in planning with patients the steps they need to take in order to regain/retain their health. The Wholistic Health Center staff attempts to take seriously the wholeness of the person, in health or disease, and offer treatment accordingly.

Whether patients come in pain or for a routine physical checkup, they find at the Wholistic Health Centers that our physicians and nurses allow time to listen carefully to their concerns and keep them informed about their findings and interpretations. Out of a sensitivity to the whole person, the Wholistic Health Centers make it possible for people to have someone to talk to for periods of time more extended than a physician or nurse can ordinarily allow.

If people come to explore problems of the human spirit, a Wholistic Health Center counselor will not moralize or try to convert them to a particular religious belief. He/she will listen with understanding and help them to discover a sense of their own worth, support them in a crisis situation, and clarify their strengths and values, including the ultimate values that make life worth living.

On the first visit, patients are asked to participate in an Initial Health Planning Conference involving the nurse, physician, and pastoral counselor. In preparation for this meeting, the patient completes a Personal Health Inventory, indicating his/her physical symptoms, emotional symptoms, goals for change, personal strengths and assets, and the kinds of help needed/requested. In addition, the individual completes a checklist of changes that have occurred for him/her during the past few years.

When the patient arrives for the appointment, the nurse registers height, weight, blood pressure, and the significant medical history; then the Planning Conference begins. The patient describes the problem; the nurse, pastor, and physician help to explore aspects of the problem and its affect on the total health of the individual. Finally, together with the patient as a team member and active participant, the team decides on a plan for further diagnosis and/or treatment as necessary and desired.

Although the treatment responsibility may be assigned to one staff member, the rest of the team stays in touch through periodic update conferences. The staff is continually on the lookout for strengths in the patient that may be tapped for creative, nontraditional treatment approaches. The Initial Health Planning Conference is described in detail in Chapter 7.

## THE PATIENTS

Who comes to the Centers? Most people first hear about us from former patients who continue to be our biggest source of referral. Others hear a speech, attend a stress course, see a notice in the church bulletin, or read about us in the newspaper. Some are referred by physicians, others by their pastor or a local counselor, and still others by the school system.

The patients are old or young, children, adolescents, college students, poverty stricken, or upper-middle class. They come as individuals, couples, families.

People come with sore throats, financial worries, inability to concentrate, broken bones, headaches, flu, ulcers, fear of failure, doubts about faith, inability to get along with the boss, pin worms, strep throat, high blood pressure, alcoholism, depression, "nerves," lacerated fingers, chest pains, low self-confidence, marital tension, warts, arthritis, multiple sclerosis, anger at parents, desire to make better decisions, for health checkups, to quit smoking, to improve the family communication, to work out an exercise program. Some come for illness care, others to improve their health, others to change their style of living. They come for colitis, grief over a friend's death, and for backaches. The point is that people come to the Wholistic Health Center for the full range of personal health concerns in which we human beings seem to be good at getting ourselves trapped.

The Wholistic Health Centers are places in which the whole person is invited to be actively engaged in the process of becoming and staying healthy—the process of taking care of himself/herself.

Some need laboratory tests for further diagnosis; others need someone to listen to their feelings. Some need encouragement; others need a swift kick. Some need surgery; others need to cut out their focus on the past and live in the present. Some need to make commitments; others need to say "no" and get out from under some pressing demands. Whatever they need, we try very hard to listen carefully and respond.

Almost anybody comes, from almost every imaginable referral source, for almost every kind of problem, and they get a wide variety of treatments. But they always get time to be heard and a wholistic approach to their concerns.

## SUMMARY

The Wholistic Health Centers, therefore, offer services similar to health services offered at other clinics on the one hand. On the other hand, the Wholistic Health Center offers something very unique.

Wholistic care at the centers utilizes a very unlikely combination of services that are unwieldy, ungainly, difficult to coordinate. Yet the concept of whole-person care is an idea whose time has come; it is perhaps the most natural and commonsense combination of talents, helpers, and settings to be found in American health care today.

Practicing health care in the Wholistic Health Centers means some very simple yet fundamental changes from today's usual style of practice. It means bringing a wide variety of resources together for the patient in one location and on one team. It means working with and appreciating other professionals with totally different training approaches and expertise. It means slowing down enough to take time to listen. It means looking for how a disease, any disease, affects the total person. It means respecting other people—the patients—as responsible adults, able to care for themselves.

Wholistic health care is obvious, yet sometimes hard to understand or accept. It is just that simple—and that difficult.

## Chapter 6

# THE WHOLISTIC HEALTH CENTER PHILOSOPHY

The efforts of the Center staff are based on a set of beliefs that gives meaning and direction to the care methodologies (diagnostic, planning, treatment, and educational activities) that are characteristic of the Centers. Ten beliefs, considered central to the practice of wholistic health care, have been isolated in the continuing development of wholistic philosophy as practiced in the Wholistic Health Centers (Tubesing, 1977).

1. *We believe that primary health care should be conveniently available to all; that the delivery of care should be structured for the convenience of the patient instead of the providers.*

The decrease in primary care physicians and the increase in centralization of services has caused long waiting periods in offices, delays in getting appointments, long commutes to the physician's office, and the need to take off significant work time to obtain health care.

The Wholistic Health Centers are located in neighborhood churches, as close to the population they serve as possible. Hours are flexible, with some evening and Saturday times available. Each Center limits its patient load so that waiting times and appointment delays are kept to a minimum. It is intended that no Center will be allowed to grow beyond an as yet undefined maximum patient load. When the maximum is reached, another staff can be recruited and a Center started nearby.

2. *We believe that health care should be focused as much as possible on the promotion of health in its broadest sense, instead of on the curing of only physical illness; correspondingly, we believe that health teams should focus on the process of keeping people healthy instead of entirely on crisis care for sicknesses.*

"Health" services are not incorporated into most primary health care offices. If you get an appointment and aren't sick, you either get a physical examination or nothing at all.

We have seen that persons who could be classified as "worried well" are in need of an increasing amount of the providers' time and energy. By conservative estimates, the majority of the sick population is in the early stages of illness; yet little or no professional care is available to focus on the early problems and on prevention of a major illness. As discussed in Chapter 2, both providers and consumers are caught in a nonproductive cycle: providers have barely enough time and energy to meet the constant demands for crisis care, while consumers get little attention unless they convince themselves and their physicians that the ailment is of crisis proportions.

The Wholistic Health Centers provide an entry into the health care system for persons who "just aren't feeling well," but do not yet feel they are sick and, therefore, would not seek regular medical care. The Initial Health Planning Conference outlines the context for this health exploration. The Conference also helps the staff to recognize those people who seek medical care mainly because they are lonely and need contact with another person, and allows the staff the opportunity to offer them contact with and attention from persons other than the physician. Patients are encouraged to come in periodically to "plan for their health" and to take stock of their health behaviors before they get sick.

3. *We believe that the focus of any plan for treatment or prevention must recognize and respect the whole person.*

The relationship between stress caused by life changes and the onset of illness is today widely accepted as fact. Nonetheless, while stress is recognized as a basic component in the development of illness, this knowledge is rarely used in typical treatment modalities.

Modern medicine emphasizes physical healing, largely disregarding the emotional and spiritual factors of the individual—factors that have been documented by the medical profession itself to have significant effect on the onset and outcome of physical illness.

The thought pattern of "divide into small pieces," of knowledge, specialize, and conquer, has produced a high level of technical knowledge but has fragmented and compartmentalized the whole person. The traditional health care system doesn't consider the whole person.

At the Centers, the skills of clergy-counselors with specialized training in grief and personal adjustment counseling are utilized to assist highly stressed persons in making sensible life-style decisions. In this way, the staff attempts to prevent the onset of additional illness. In addition, creative treatment plans attempt to utilize patient strengths drawing from all aspects of life. The centers do not emphasize "yearly physical exams"; we provide instead "annual Health Planning Conferences" that examine the intellectual, social, emotional, and spiritual aspects of health as well as the physical aspect.

Regular courses such as "The Creative Management of Stress" are attempts to teach our patients the wholistic view of health and to stimulate them to take better care of themselves.

*4. We believe that wholistic health care is practiced most effec-
tively by a team of professionals each with different personalities and
different training experiences.*

Wholistic health care is simply beyond the ability of
any one provider, no matter how well trained. One person
cannot gain all of the knowledge and skills necessary for
treatment within the wholistic context. No matter how
emotionally healthy the provider, he/she cannot expect to
feel comfortable and build trust with every patient, nor can
one provider accurately process all of the verbal and nonverbal communications of every patient all of the time.
When professionals work as a team, both the professional
knowledge and personal "gut level" reactions of each team
member can, when pooled, result in a diagnosis and treatment plan much more likely to be focused on the central
problem of the patient. In a team context, physicians are
not required to treat problems that are related to emotional
or social causes, and counselors are not asked to diagnose
and treat diseases that are related to physical causes.

The teamwork of a widely diverse interdisciplinary
staff is one of the core elements of wholistic care as practiced within the Wholistic Health Centers.

*5. We believe the patient is a responsible adult, capable of
contributing to his/her own diagnosis and treatment, and should be
considered an active participant on the health care team.*

Too often patients are treated like children who
"wouldn't understand." Too often patients accept the passive role and fail to act in their own behalf.

In the Wholistic Health Centers, the patient is expected to participate actively in decisions concerning treatment. The patient, not the staff, "owns" the information
about his/her case. The charts are open for the patient's
viewing. At times, patients make new entries or correct
previous entries on the charts. Life-style and behavior decisions, considered essential in the recovery and maintenance of health, are in full control of the patient and are
acknowledged as such. When no absolute answers are

available, the staff presents alternatives for the patient's consideration and/or decision.

6. *We believe that health education and health screening programs are essential health service functions of a primary health care facility.*

Patient education programs need to emphasize the wholistic instead of the partistic nature of personal health and to encourage the development of healthy life-styles that may prevent the onset of some illness and will lead to more personal satisfaction in life. Greater emphasis on education for illness prevention should, in the long run, prove to be more economical than our present crisis care (reactive) system. It should be less expensive to educate people concerning detection, diagnosis, and management of certain diseases than to care for those who become disabled and economically unproductive as a consequence of the disease.

The Centers are attempting to reach the healthy population before people get sick and are attempting to involve persons in health education and preventive screening programs such as: (a) a series of health seminars (including the creative management of grief and stress, healthy dynamics of family life, first aid, etc.); (b) the formation of personal support groups (focusing on weight loss, stopping smoking, and assertiveness); and (c) community health fairs. The focus of these programs is behavior change and decision making, not mere information imparting.

7. *We believe that when more than one provider is "treating a person," the coordination of care and the communication of information between the variety of professionals is essential to the wellbeing of the individual patient.*

The hazards to a patient who sees four or five different specialists, each of whom may be recommending different and incompatible types of medication or treatment, are widely recognized. Normally, patients who see several specialists are forced to spend a great deal of energy and must possess substantial expertise in order to coordinate the variety of treatments they may be receiving. Unfortunately, wholistic health care is the exception; fragmented treatment is the rule.

Family physicians, with their emphasis on primary care and family medicine, are particularly sensitive to this issue of rational coordination of an individual's health care. The fact that the family practice specialty appears to be a genuine and growing force in this country is comforting. When personal disease, however, is considered within the context of the whole person (physical, emotional, social, intellectual, and spiritual), the need for an even wider coordination between medical, religious, counseling, and social service professionals becomes evident.

The teamwork concept of the Centers focuses on coordination of a wholistic form of care and allows the expertise of various professionals to be brought to bear on an individual's health problems. When making either counseling or medical referrals to specialists outside the Centers, special effort is expended to gather and integrate care reports and to interpret the data to the patient in a manner that is understandable to him/her.

8. *We believe that it is the responsibility of the health care providers to offer the greatest possible service for each dollar expended.*

The increased cost of both hospital and ambulatory care in the United States is presently decried by both providers and patients. However, huge capital expenditures are still being invested for new buildings and duplicate services.

The Wholistic Health Center staff works on a salary— a reasonable, livable salary. The church location of the Centers provide free space with essentially no overhead expenses and almost no capital investment. In addition, the use of professional and paraprofessional volunteers and the concept of allowing people (patients) to help each other assist the staff in providing greater quality care for less dollar expenditure.

9. *We believe that our communities, and particularly churches, abound with talented people who desire the opportunity to volunteer their time and skill in helping others.*

Few health care facilities have managed to tap the great potential resource of auxiliary paraprofessional healing agents who could lighten the burden of providers and supply some of the contact services needed by persons who are concerned about their health.

The Wholistic Health Centers are testing out new ideas for recruiting and utilizing the skills of a variety of volunteer workers. The paid staff members multiply their time about 100% by involving volunteers in the patient care and health education activities of each local Center.

10. *We believe that the essential processes operating within a healing relationship are qualities that every human being possesses. People can be helpful to each other.*

Traditional forms of primary medical care have been limited mainly to interactions between the health care professional and the patient. The extreme shortage of medical professionals has become a powerful force in stimulating the search for more efficient means of expanding the professional resources. In the wider scope of wholistic and preventive health care, other models must be developed that will utilize volunteer professionals, paraprofessionals, and patient support groups.

Support services are needed now more than ever, since the institutions that once provided support at times of transition (birth, death, and crisis) are diminishing rapidly. The extended family is vanishing; the church is less potent; neighbors are less helpful; and social casework services are insufficient.

The Centers attempt to mobilize the multitude of "people helping people" health resources within the local church communities and bring them to bear on individual and community health problems. A list is kept of local interest groups, educational opportunities, and so on. Persons are often referred to these as part of their treatment plan. In addition to patient support groups focused on various problems, one patient may be put in contact with another patient who has experienced similar health difficulties and is learning to cope creatively. At times such contacts have been at least as helpful as any professional-patient contact experienced at the Center.

## SUMMARY

The needs in the present system are a catalyst to the establishment and testing of innovative models for the delivery of primary health care in the country. The 10 beliefs in the Wholistic Health Centers' "creed" have been the guideposts in the formulation of patient care procedures at the Centers. The process of enacting these beliefs is, of course, continually in the stage of development.

The following chapters detail present methodologies for enacting these beliefs.

## Chapter 7

# INTRODUCING THE PATIENT TO THE WHOLISTIC HEALTH CENTER PROCESS

The keystone of the care methodology as now practiced in the Wholistic Health Centers is the Initial Health Planning Conference: a 20-minute joint "intake" session attended by the patient, the nurse, the physician, and the director of counseling, who "chairs" the session.

The Initial Health Planning Conference is the heart of the patient care offered in the Wholistic Health Centers. It sets them apart from other attempts at comprehensive health care by their emphasis on the interdisciplinary team-work approach, their focus on planning and prevention, and the involvement of patients as responsible adults, active in the management of their own health.[1]

[1] Peterson et al., 1976

## THE INITIAL HEALTH PLANNING CONFERENCE
### (Peterson et al., 1976)

### AN OVERVIEW

Under normal circumstances patients participate in a Health Planning Conference during their first Center visit. The people complete a Personal Health Inventory (PHI) modified from Holmes and Rahe's Social Readjustment Rating Scale (Holmes & Rahe, 1967). The complete form is reproduced in Figure 7.1. When possible, the patients complete this inventory before coming for the first appointment. The PHI is designed to help people to recognize the variety of stress factors at work in their lives at the moment, focus on a definition of the problem, list their resources and strengths, and isolate the areas in which they desire professional help in moving toward health.

The Center nurse, whose role is that of patient advocate both in the Conference and for follow-up appointments, meets with patients individually in an adjoining office, getting acquainted while recording vital medical signs. A brief history is taken at this time to begin assembling patient files. The nurse and the patient then join the physician and the director of counseling for the Health Planning Conference. The counselor briefly describes the Wholistic Health Center philosophy and the purpose of the Planning Conference, and asks patients what brings them to the Center. The patients are encouraged to discuss all dimensions of life affected by the disease that they are experiencing. The staff members help the patients to explore related aspects revealed by the health inventory. This listening, clarifying, summarizing activity focused on defining the problem is the activity that demands the most time, energy, and attention in the Conference. Following the problem definition phase, staff members give patients

## PERSONAL HEALTH INVENTORY

Welcome to the Wholistic Health Center.

Our intention in your first visit is to engage you in an individualized plan for becoming and staying healthy. We believe that being healthy is more than having a body that works well; it is feeling good about yourself, dealing creatively with the people and situations around you, and growing spiritually toward a sense of wholeness.

In our initial planning conference, you will meet with a health care team consisting of a physician, nurse, and director of counseling. We'll talk together about which of our professional skills would be most helpful to you and arrive at a plan for working together. We recognize that the final decisions about the plan are up to you; the best we can do is make recommendations and offer our services.

We've found that people appreciate and benefit from an opportunity to reflect on all of their concerns prior to the initial conference. This pamphlet is offered as a tool to help focus your reflections before the planning conference. Please bring it with you.

If you have any questions about this pamphlet or the conference, please ask any of the staff. We appreciate your comments.

**Figure 7.1   The Personal Health Inventory**

Your Name: _____ Date: _____

**I. Physical symptoms I'm concerned about:**

_____

_____

_____

_____

**II. Life Change Checklist**[*]

Check events which have occured in the past few years and circle those that have been most stressful. Reflect on these changes before completing the remainder of the inventory.

PERSONAL EVENTS AND CHANGES

_____ Death of a close friend or family member

_____ Personal injury, illness, or hospitalization

_____ Pregnancy (or pregnancy of spouse)

_____ Loss of self confidence

_____ Outstanding achievement (graduation, promotion)

_____ Change in eating habits

_____ Change in sexual activity

_____ Change in sleeping patterns

_____ Change in energy level

_____ Considered suicide

_____ Change in religious belief or practice

_____ Stress related to vacation

_____ Change in relationship with parents

_____ Change in recreational time/activity

[*]Adapted from the work of Thomas Holmes, M.D., University of Washington.

_____ Trouble with the law

_____ Change in time schedule

Change in _____ drinking _____ smoking _____ drug use

Other: _____

## CHANGES IN MARITAL RELATIONSHIP

_____ Married _____ Divorced _____ Separated

_____ Living Together

_____ Disagreements over money management

_____ Increased emotional distance

_____ Trouble with in-laws

_____ Spouse beginning or stopping work or school

Other: _____

## CHANGES IN THE HOUSEHOLD

_____ Family member left home

_____ Gain of a new member (birth, parents moving in, adoption, etc.)

_____ Spouse at home more than before

_____ Problems with children at home

_____ Change in residence

_____ Remodeling or building

_____ Change in health/behavior/attitude of a member of the household

_____ Change in neighbors or neighborhood

Other: _____

## CHANGES AT WORK

_____ New job, or new line of work

_____ Quit _____ Fired _____ Retired _____ Laid Off

_____ Less job security

_____ Promotion _____ Demotion

_____ Trouble with work associates

_____ Change in hours, conditions, travel, etc.

Other: _____


## FINANCIAL CHANGES

_____ Changes in financial state (better or worse)

_____ Major mortgage or loan taken out

_____ Foreclosure of mortgage or loan

Other: _____

_____


III. Feelings/emotions I'm concerned about:

_____

_____

_____

_____


IV. Goals toward which I'd like to begin moving:

_____

_____

_____

_____


V. My strong points and special abilities in moving toward my goals:

_____

_____

_____

_____


VI. Kinds of help I need in moving toward my goals:

some feedback on resources, test procedures, and ways of beginning to deal with the concerns raised. Patients participate actively in deciding the final diagnosis and course of treatment. Fees for the planned treatment are discussed. Immediate care may be given, if necessary, or the nurse assists patients in making arrangements and appointments for treatment at future dates. When appropriate, referral to a specialist is initiated.

Sometimes the Planning Conference focuses on acute illness (e.g., URI, injury) or extreme emotional distress (e.g., depression, marital strife) that needs immediate treatment. At these times, appropriate medical and/or psychological diagnosis and care is immediately initiated, and a plan is established for continued care. At other times, however (e.g., general checkup), the Conference focuses on assisting people in the formation of a plan of action for maintaining health and preventing disease. When this is the focus, attention is given to affirming positive health behaviors and acknowledging personal strengths and resources, as well as isolating potential problem areas.

Whether it is focused on an acute health problem or on prevention and health maintenance, the Conference, almost without exception, proves to be worthwhile in terms of clarifying problems, focusing on new behaviors, and helping people to establish a plan for treatment and health maintenance that will be effective for and agreeable to them. Patients are considered the experts on the kind of help they want at the moment. Their knowledge is respected in the treatment planning process, as the staff works to understand the values, sense of rhythm, and expressed needs of patients.

Often patients revise their initial analysis of the problem as the Conference progresses. If a simple acute medical problem is prominent, the staff may ask, "Do the areas of stress noted on your inventory affect your physical health as you see it?" If the problem appears to call for counseling alone, the staff may ask, "How is this emotional/social stress affecting you physically?" Commonly, the staff finds that the presenting symptoms can be handled quite easily, while the underlying problem is more difficult to define and requires more skillful treatment and extensive care before it is rectified. Sometimes, the "mere" redefinition of the problem acts as a treatment and provides an immediate and obvious solution.

Following the Initial Health Planning Conference, patients return to the Center for counseling care, medical care, or health education consultation with individual staff members, as needed. During most of these individual problem-focused care encounters, patients meet with either the pastoral counselor, the physician, or the nurse, and care is delivered in a manner similar to that of more traditional counseling or medical treatment facilities. However, crossover, coordinated care can occur at any time during treatment, when either patients or providers see the need.

## MANAGING THE PLANNING CONFERENCE

The Health Planning Conference is designed as an assessment and planning meeting, not as a counseling session or a medical examination period. Of course, in the clarification of the problem, the teaching, the listening, and the personal contact during the Conference, treatment is already going on. In a sense, treatment begins at the moment people first call for an appointment.

### Defining the Problem

During the problem-definition phase of the Conference, people are encouraged to discuss their concerns and explore all dimensions of life affected by the disease they are experiencing. Staff members help patients to explore the physical, emotional, life-style, interpersonal, and spiritual dimensions of the problem they bring. The definition of the problem is really a "history taking" in all areas of health. The staff actively listens for patterns of health and disease and investigates relationships between the physical and other dimensions of health.

Special focus is placed on identifying needs for which patients want help and in clarifying the resources that people already have for dealing with the problem. In describing their strengths, patients can teach the staff a lot about their coping abilities. The staff can, in return, reinforce and support patients in activating those resources in their life. In addition to encouraging people to look at their inner resources, the staff team helps them to clarify what they can change and what they cannot change.

*Clarifying the Problem*

The problem-clarification phase of the Health Planning Conference is the most difficult to manage. The format is unstructured. The direction and flow depend on the concerns that patients bring with them.

People usually select one of the three staff members with whom they talk most directly during the Conference. Most often they choose the pastoral director, but they may choose the doctor or the nurse. The chosen staff member manages the flow of the conversation, with the other staff members breaking in as little as possible.

During this part of the Conference, the staff's ability to communicate and work together is tested. There must be an almost intuitive sense of timing among staff members about who wants to talk next and the direction of movement with different patients.

The staff decides together how the Planning Conference time is to be spent. The three staff members may find themselves each wanting to explore different areas. If this happens, the best way we have found for handling the difficulty seems to be by expressing the conflict openly and freely. This communication among staff members in front of patients demonstrates the teamwork concept and our willingness to include them in the process.

Discussion and clarification of the problem demands the most attentive, careful listening by the staff. This listening, clarifying, and summarizing actually comprises the majority of time in the Conference.

When the problem is defined as clearly as possible, each staff member gives feedback by sharing with the patient possible resources, test procedures, or ways of beginning to tackle the concerns that have been raised.

*Treatment Planning*

Planning for treatment begins with the question, "Given all these concerns, what do you need to do to take care of yourself?" This is often a highly emotional point in the Conference, as people begin to think of long-delayed decisions or are astounded at the expectation that they take care of themselves.

People frequently *do* know what they need to do to take care of themselves. Unfortunately, health care providers rarely ask this crucial question. People may not know all the technical, medical, or therapeutic kinds of language to go along with it, but they do know whether they need to sit down with a counselor and sort some things out, whether they need some kinds of medical help, or whether they need a good vacation.

Questions like this engage people in thinking about and making their own decisions for their own health care. If people obviously need to make a number of different changes in order to care for themselves, this is the time in the Conference when priorities for care are established, recognizing that everything cannot be done at once.

Together the team members (including the patients) come up with a specific plan of care for the concerns raised.

In designing the plan, the team considers the needs of the patients, the importance of further exploration of staff observations and assessments, and the readiness of people to engage in different kinds of decision making.

Patients are involved in selecting their plan for treatment. They are encouraged to express their reactions and can rule out any plans that they would not accept or carry out. The physician, nurse, and counselor are experts in knowing the kinds of help they have to offer. They make their ideas, concerns, and limitations known to patients. Patients are the experts on their own problems. People know what kind of help they want at this time. This knowledge is respected in the planning process.

The staff works to respect the values and the sense of rhythm and timing of the patient. Is now the time to tackle the problem at its root, or just do a "patch job" for a while? The patient decides.

Sometimes, although wholeness in health is a goal, patients need to keep some pieces of their lives separate and not integrated. At other times, patients need to lean on someone and be dependent for awhile. These can be temporary and acceptable ways for getting through crises.

Patients also choose their own pace for moving toward health. Perhaps they don't want to start exercising, stop eating eggs, stop drinking alcohol, and stop smoking all in one day. People have a right to choose how much they want to do at any one time.

We try not to impose our standards on the patient. The question about treatment is put to the patient. "Is this a big enough problem in your life, that you want us to help you work on it now?"

The staff works hard at clarifying mutual assumptions, checking them out, and establishing a clear "contract" for expectations of each other—at getting the decision clearly stated.

### REFLECTIONS ON THE PLANNING CONFERENCE

The preceding section tells the story of "how we do it." This section focuses on some of the rationale for "why we do what we do," and presents some observations on the Conference.

First, we consider two pillars of the Health Planning Conference: the treatment of patients as adults and the Personal Health Inventory. Next, we look at some variations on the Initial Health Planning Conference for persons with special needs. Finally, we view once again the overall picture of the Conference, set it in context, and point out some advantages for using this format as a major treatment modality.

### Patients as Adults

People who come to the Wholistic Health Center for care are treated as competent adults, capable of caring for a majority of their own health needs. From the initial contact with the secretary/receptionist, through the steps of the Initial Health Planning Conference, to the completion of the treatment plan, Center staff members expend the greatest part of their effort on assisting and educating patients to mobilize their resources for health.

During the Planning Conference, patients are active participants on the healing team. Their expertise, their knowledge of the problem, and their ideas for a workable treatment plan are a major contribution to the Conference. As members of their own healing teams, patients are often knowledgeable about possible causes and possible cures. Motivation for change comes from the patients, not the providers.

We ask patients to choose their own treatment plans, encourage them to consider and identify ways they might normally sabotage such a plan, and challenge them to design strategies to safeguard themselves against their own subtle setups for failure.

Most people handle nearly all day-to-day problems with their own resources. They need help only when their natural healthy coping resources and mechanisms are temporarily not maintaining their health. At the Centers, the goal is to reinforce their resources through short-range, long-range, or total life-style planning, so they can begin to take care of themselves more fully again.

One of the most innovative ways that we seek to affirm the response-ability and maturity of people who seek care at the Centers is through our policy of "patient ownership" of medical records. Many people are surprised by the freedom they have to read staff notes on their progress and even to make entries in their own charts. If patients are going to transfer records from another health care provider, that provider is also told about our open records policy.

## Personal Health Inventory

The Personal Health Inventory (PHI) that people complete prior to the Health Planning Conference helps individuals to recognize the variety of stress factors at work in their lives, focus on a definition of the problem, list their resources and strengths, and isolate the areas where they desire professional help in moving toward health. The PHI is designed more for preparing patients for the Planning Conference and teaching them to look at the wholeness of their health than it is for professional diganostic use. However, the PHI is a very effective "discussion prodder" in the Conference itself.

People often check items on the PHI that they want to talk about, but have difficulty bringing up. We try to be sensitive to what people leave out in their problem presentation as well as the concerns that they verbalize. The counseling director may ease the way for people by saying,

> I see you've checked 'small children at home' on your life change inventory, but haven't mentioned any concerns in that area with us. Does this stress fit in with the rest of the things we've been talking about?

This question gives people permission to explore concerns that they may have been afraid to share, or it may call their attention to areas of stress they had not considered particularly important before.

The PHI also includes space for recording significant achievements on the path to more healthy living. Patients can affirm their growth as the treatment plan is carried out.

The use of the PHI in our care methodology is based on three convictions: (1) stress is a causal factor in disease; (2) identifying both needs and resources is in itself therapeutic for the patient; and (3) the process of identifying recent life stresses teaches patients a method for analyzing their personal disease in the future.

### Variations on the Initial Health Planning Conference

The structure of the Planning Conference is flexible enough to adapt to the specific needs of different persons.

ACUTE PROBLEMS.    If people have an acute illness or an acute counseling problem, the Planning Conference will be shortened and we will proceed to treatment in the first visit. If people are in crisis, the Conference is delayed until a later date. Most people who come to the Center, however, do not need immediate care for extensive problems.

REQUESTS FOR MEDICAL TREATMENT ONLY.    When people come to the Center for medical reasons, and if their PHI does not indicate substantial life changes or emotional problems, the pastoral director may say:

> It sounds like you're here primarily for medical care. If you're also interested in counseling, or if you wish to ask me any questions, I don't want to miss that.

People at this point can indicate whether or not they want to talk with the pastoral counselor. If they indicate they did not come for counseling and want medical care only, the pastoral counselor says:

> I am available for consultation if you have any questions where I might be helpful. I don't engage everybody in long-term therapy; in fact, most of the counseling that we do here is relatively short-term. Many people choose to see a counselor for one or two sessions just to sort something out, and I'm available for that now or any time in the future.

He/she may describe preventive education programs offered by the Center that are of potential interest, talk about fees, and discuss the open chart policy. The pastoral director then leaves the Conference. The nurse and physician attend to the immediate physical concerns and may schedule further examination and additional procedures as needed.

*REQUEST FOR COUNSELING SERVICES ONLY.*        If it is clear that patients have come exclusively for counseling services and not for medical care, the physician (about 10 minutes into the Conference) may say:

> I hear that you are here primarily for counseling, but if you are seeking medical care I don't want to miss that.

Patients at this point indicate whether they have any questions about their physical health and whether they are under the care of another physician.

Occasionally patients do have some questions to ask the physician, questions that have been put off because they felt other physicians didn't have the time to answer them. Patients may have some questions about the medication they are taking, such as what it does and what it's for. Many people who come to the Center are taking medication for which they don't understand the primary intention or the possible side effects. One patient, for example, thought Valium was something like Tums, to be taken for an upset stomach. The doctor answers any questions people may have and then says:

> I am a family physician, and I am available should you want to consult with me at any point.

The doctor then leaves the Conference.

When the staff members leave the Planning Conference, they shake hands with people, let them know it was good to meet them, and tell them once again of the availability of their services. If people come with both physical symptoms and emotional distress (the majority of cases), all staff members stay throughout the Conference.

*PREVENTIVE HEALTH PLANNING.*    When people come to the Center for preventive health planning (perhaps at the time of an annual health checkup) and have no immediate concerns (an unusual situation), we try to focus on the strengths in their current life-style. We reinforce the choices they are presently making as they cope with stress and attempt to stay creative and "alive." Sometimes we ask about the fact that no life change items have been checked on the PHI. We may need to encourage people who have stagnated to change some aspects of their life.

*Getting Out of the Way*

As people start to take active care of themselves, they have less need for our resources. When the treatment plan has been carried out, when people seem to be pretty well on their way toward a more healthy life-style, or when people are feeling better about themselves, the staff begins to step out of the way. We encourage people to rely on their own resources and let them know that we will be back in contact within the next year to schedule a brief reevaluation.

People are very appreciative when we call at different times during the year. A quick checkup phone call seems to communicate that the staff cares about them and feels that their health is important. A phone call is often enough to encourage people to stay on their program of taking care of themselves.

*Follow-up*

If people haven't been to the Center for a year or so, we will generally invite them back for another Health Planning Conference similar to the one described here, except that the history-taking is not quite so extensive. The Health Planning Conference in some ways replaces the annual physical. At this annual Conference, people reflect on issues of concern to their overall health. If there are no physical problems, we spend the time talking with people about their life-style and their health habits. At this time we also explore with people the stresses in their lives and their successful coping strategies.

## SUMMARY

The Initial Health Planning Conference is the methodology used at Wholistic Health Centers to introduce patients to wholistic health care and to engage them in the process of becoming healthy and taking care of themselves. It is quite openly an attempt to get people to do some thinking about their own health care and to begin making their own decisions.

After people are engaged as patients at the Center, the Conference is used to help people to reflect on their life-styles and to encourage them to continue taking care of themselves. The Planning Conference can also be a time to evaluate progress or to make new decisions about the treatment plan.

From a staff viewpoint, almost without exception, the Conference proves to be worthwhile in terms of clarifying problems, focusing on new behaviors, and setting out a plan for treatment agreeable to all, including the patient. The Planning Conference helps the staff to get a clear idea of what it is the patient wants from us, and how we can best proceed toward meeting those needs.

Several noteworthy advantages of the team planning approach are evident in the Initial Health Planning Conference.

> Patients become acquainted with the array of staff resources available and begin a relationship with all three staff members representing different disciplines.

> Patients are not merely told, "Your health concerns involve your whole person," but they actively live through a demonstration of that philosophy in the teamwork activity of the Conference. Often people fail to hear what is said, but seldom do they miss the message of the teamwork approach that they experience. The Initial Health Planning Conference actually turns out to be a health education program in which patients learn to understand what makes them ill and how to plan and care for themselves better.

> The expertise of patients, their knowledge of the problem, and their ideas for workable treatment plans are utilized. Patients become active participants, often lending extremely valuable analysis.

Patients are involved in selecting the plans for treatment. Patients are encouraged to express their reactions and can rule out plans that they would not accept.

The coordination of staff expertise adds a multitude of differing perspectives, which sometimes results in a richness of creative insight regarding diagnosis and treatment seldom experienced in a one-to-one treatment approach. As the staff has learned to trust and respect one another, each has learned from the others' unique professional training and personal sensitivities.

Prior to the establishment of the Initial Health Planning Conference as a regular feature of the Wholistic Health Centers' care, the staff needed (1) a way of establishing a relationship with people, setting up files, and clarifying mutual expectations; (2) a way of helping people to experience the wholistic approach to their concerns; (3) a way of eliciting the patients' participation in caring for themselves; (4) a way of carefully diagnosing problems and formulating treatment plans before proceeding to treatment; and (5) a way of managing the team's schedule efficiently. The Initial Health Planning Conference is the mechanism that currently meets these needs.

One of the chief tasks now is to prove that this multi-disciplinary approach is not only helpful in whole-person care, but that it is also economically feasible. The goal is to show that, although it is an expensive process, in the long run the Initial Health Planning Conference improves the quality of care and its consequent effect on patient health, and that it is therefore a uniquely worthwhile investment.

## Chapter 8

# THE PROFESSIONS
# RE-EXAMINED IN RELATION TO
# THE WHOLISTIC HEALTH
# CENTER

In a Center like ours, as in any human service business, it is not the plans, procedures, or philosophy that determine patients' experience; instead, it is the staff, their personalities, personal character, and the manner in which they relate to the patients. Do we care? Will we listen? Are we relaxed? Are we attentive, or are our minds elsewhere? Are we more interested in facts or feelings? The answers to these questions determine the "human spirit" quality of our care. Patients make their own judgments and answer these questions about us for themselves.

## TEAMWORK ISSUES

In staffing the clinics we look not only for persons with professional skills and academic backgrounds that would qualify them to teach graduate courses within the Centers; in addition, we need people who:

127

Can fit in with the whole person philosophy of the Center and can listen well and communicate warmth.

Want to work on a team and can blend their skills with those of the other team members.

Can manage many different tasks and delegate tasks to a corps of volunteers whom they supervise and whose efforts they coordinate.

It is a demanding job and is somewhat broader in scope than most of us received training for in our highly specialized graduate programs. It is also a lot more rewarding for us than it would be to practice only our specialty in isolation. We've learned a lot from each other.

Our learning together to work with each other for the health of the patient has occurred through many types of interaction, including health planning conferences, staff meetings, educational workshops, and informal discussions. It is within these contexts that we have struggled and worked through frustrations as we sought to develop a team. Teamwork and cooperation among a treatment team does not necessarily occur spontaneously without any attention. It must be worked at and attended to.

For instance, at first we approached our intake team conference with the total focus on patient care and our common concern for taking the whole person seriously. We were not so worried about the intrateam dynamics. In fact, as long as each professional discipline was represented, we mixed staff persons almost at random. This total lack of attention to building the team into a working unit, although well motivated since our attention was on the patient, was also naive.

Through experience we learned that this random mix of paid and volunteer staff did not allow the teamwork coordination to develop adequately. Everyone (physicians, nurses, and pastoral counselors) experienced difficulties when being "plugged into" the team without much warning or team process time. All were excellent, skilled professional people, used to working by themselves. We learned that the issues of working as a team require some time for people to become acquainted with each other, learn each other's styles, be able to sense where the others are going, and learn what issues the others will attend to. Being part of a team required development of a sense of what one has to contribute and the security of belonging, which allows each member to be active at some times and silent at others.

Since the early days, we have worked hard among our staff to build up group cohesion and mutual trust and to cut down "territorial imperialism." We have learned to blend the art of personal support with the science of diagnosis and treatment. We have continually learned from each other and grown to appreciate the others' professional expertise and personal qualities. The experience of teamwork has reinforced our belief that the planning for the treatment of health problems can best be done by an interdisciplinary team.

On the other hand, we have learned that not all patients require all of our services all at the same time, and that not all treatment needs to be done as a team. Togetherness in diagnosis and planning and in follow-up consultation is effective. Constant togetherness in carrying out the treatment as planned is seldom necessary and questionably effective.

## The Professions Revisited

Combining the unique professional skills contributed by each discipline and blending the roles and the planning of treatment approaches that cross over normal professional interest lines is at the heart of the health care we offer to each other and to our patients.

The role tasks and job description for each professional within the Wholistic Health Center context are presented below. The focus has been placed on comparing the professional activities within the teamwork practiced in the Center with the activities that would be considered normal for the profession in a more traditional setting.

## The Role of the Nurse

Is our nurse an emergency room nurse? A psychiatric nurse? A visiting nurse? A staff supervising nurse? A public health nurse? A nurse clinician? An in-service educator? A team leader? A nurse practitioner? The answer is "Yes." All these facets of nursing duties and skills are called for in the Center's routine. I've seen one of our staff nurses throw up her hands in mock helplessness when someone asked, "What is the role of the nurse?"

The nurse attends all staff conferences. She/he works with patients in direct treatment, medical exams, education and informational consultations and, at times, in counseling sessions. She/he ensures that sufficient medical supplies are on hand and monitors the charting procedures. The Wholistic Health Center nurse has a great deal of freedom to set up consultations and teaching programs with patients and to make follow-up phone calls to patients at her/his own initiative.

As the job of the Center nurse has evolved, she/he is seen serving in two distinct roles: patient advocate and coordinator of volunteers.

THE NURSE AS PATIENT ADVOCATE.    As patient advocate the nurse become the support person in the clinic for the patient. She/he greets the patient, establishes a relationship of trust, explains the Wholistic Health Center concept, prepares the patient for conferences, and gets the basic background medical information for the charts. She/he attempts to lessen the patient's anxiety by telling the patient what to expect in any treatment. She/he introduces the patient to the other staff members and facilitates communication of the patient's concerns. If the patient is dissatisfied, the nurse remains a safe person with whom the patient can share his/her complaints.

Additional aspects of the patient advocacy role are the nurse's presence during all physical examinations, responsibility for follow-up in locating resources, and explaining procedures that will be necessary for completion of the treatment plan. At times, the nurse becomes a link between the physician and the counselor, stimulating revision of treatment plans that are not working for patients.

Nurses have long been in the natural position of being patient advocates. At the Wholistic Health Center, this position of advocacy is encouraged because it is necessary to the effective practice of our style of care.

*THE NURSE AS COORDINATOR OF VOLUNTEERS.*    As coordinator of volunteers, the Center nurse recruits, trains, and supervises the work of six to eight volunteer nurses. The Center offers so many types of care-related services, no one person could accomplish them all. The numerous volunteers, each with different skills, can complement one another. The skills one lacks, another may fulfill easily. The assignment of tasks and assessment of personal skills and weaknesses is, of course, essential to the coordination of the volunteer staff of nurses.

Wholistic health care philosophy is certainly not new to nurses, although they usually have called it "comprehensive care." Beginning nursing students are taught to attend to all aspects of the patient's needs: physical, emotional, spiritual, and environmental.

Within the Wholistic Health Center context, however, a number of unique challenges are offered to the nurses. They are challenged to discover new ways to involve patients more in the team process and to explore new ways of assisting the patients to better care for their own health. Nurses are encouraged to be independent and relate as peers on the health care team. The nurses have some decision-making power concerning the care of the patient.

In the Center both physicians and counselors have repeatedly stated that they appreciate the value of the nurse's contribution to team discussions and her/his ability to deal with people who are in emotional or physical pain. One of our physicians commented, "I think the talents of the nurse are used more effectively in the Wholistic Health Center than in any other setting I have seen."

What is it like for the nurse to work in the Wholistic Health Center? One joked when asked this question on a particularly long day: "Everyone I've seen today has to cry. I just look at them and buckets of tears start running, and then I'm listening for 20 minutes." But she wasn't complaining, because that is what her/his job in the Wholistic Health Center setting is all about.

### The Role of the Physician

The physician is a key member of the Wholistic Health Center team because everyone knows that you can't have a full-fledged health care center without a physician. One of the unique characteristics of the physicians who practice in the Wholistic Health Centers, however, is that they have been willing to give up some of the total autonomy traditionally given physicians in order to practice health care surrounded by a team and in order to be free from the trap of always having to have all of the answers all of the time. It is not uncommon for our physicians to say something like, "I don't know, but I will find out."

The Wholistic Health Center is a family practice clinic. The physicians in the Centers do everything other family practice physicians normally do. Limited laboratory tests are completed at the Center, but patients are sent to a local laboratory for extensive workups and/or X rays. Our physicians are on the staffs of local hospitals and admit patients to the hospital when necessary. Their professional growth is stimulated by consultation with specialists, interaction with medical colleagues, and continuing education seminars.

On the other hand, the family practice focus of the Centers' activities call for a physician with interests and skills beyond the technical. One of our physicians described his personal approach this way.

When I was in medical school there was always a big push for the specialties, where lots of exciting things were going on. All our training was divided up into specialties. But for me, something was lacking. How do we bring it all together? Where does disease fit into a person's life after I've given medications? How do I deal with the person . . . with the family?

So I became a family physician. In my practice I take care of the whole family. I try to do preventive medicine by sensing the problems before the breakdown occurs, by observing the little stresses in the family. I try to offer total care to the family, and I enter the family through any member and I ask, 'What are the relationships like in your family?' Sometimes I schedule time to talk to the whole family together.

I'm not here to take kids away from pediatricians. I'm not here to take women from the gynecologists. But the thing that gets the specialists excited is a rare disease in his specialty. Most specialists want to get rid of general exams. But me, I want routine care. I get excited about primary routine care. My goal is to keep people well. I don't like to see sick people, but when I have to I want the whole family behind me, and I want to know where the strengths are in that family that I can call on.

The Wholistic Health Center physicians focus not only on a disease, but on improving the total health of the patient. They deal with human concerns, not merely with disease and technological treatments. When a woman has a lump in her breast, what is the problem? Is it the lump? Is it the woman's fear? Or is it the husband's anxiety? All sensitive physicians would say, "It's all three." At the Wholistic Health Centers the resources for treating all three are immediately available.

One of the Centers' physicians who also has a private practice in a rural area compared the style of her practice in the two settings.

> In my rural practice I want to respond to the needs and concerns of my patients, not just diseases and physical symptoms, but often three things stop me: (1) I haven't the time or the energy to respond; too many others are waiting; (2) people don't feel comfortable bringing out the underlying problem; the situation isn't structured to encourage this discussion; and (3) sometimes I simply miss the problem. The difference in the Wholistic Health Center is that the structure of the Planning Conference gives patients permission to raise concerns from any area of life and I have the support staff to help them deal with the concerns in depth.

Another Center physician remarked on the uniqueness of practice in the Wholistic Health Centers.

> I prescribe less medication here, because normally I would have few options. In the Wholistic Health Center I can offer people a chance to work at the root of the problem and I can know something is being done about it.
> Along with the pastoral counselor and nurse, I struggle to find a way that you can effectively and smoothly minister to people who are in pain, in need, who are concerned about their health.
> It's a startling process to try to get people of two disciplines, counseling and medicine, to work together on an equal footing, but that's what we're struggling with.

The answers we search for may be multifaceted. They certainly are not simple. But it's a worthwhile venture, and we're on the right track.

Learning to promote positive health habits and positive addictions for people, learning to listen better, learning to hook people into taking care of themselves, and learning to ask them what plans of action they will agree to follow are among the skills our physicians have developed.

## The Role of the Pastoral Counselor

The counseling directors of the Centers are pastors (priests or rabbis) who have attained a graduate degree and certification in counseling as a social worker, psychologist, or marriage and family counselor after their seminary training.

The pastoral counselors are the Centers' administrators. They are responsible for the educational program, for supervising volunteer counselors, for calling case conferences together, and for ensuring that the philosophy of the Wholistic Health Center is activated in all phases of the Centers' operations.

The pastoral counselor is counselor, supervisor, accountant, PR director, claims adjustor, odd job expert, financial development officer, public servant, personnel officer, general contractor, and director of educational programs. These are all necessary duties that add a sense of variety and that sometimes produce the exhilaration of skirting disaster.

The pastors are not interested in proselytizing or gaining membership in any denominational church. Although all counselors have a specific content to their faith, the content is not "pushed" on the patient. Instead, the issues of faith, value, meaning, and commitment decisions in a person's life are actively considered as a legitimate aspect of health. The counselor who senses a person is having trouble with particular feelings will certainly ask, "What are you feeling?" and will help the individual sort out his/her feelings. The pastoral counselor who senses that a person is having trouble with the faith issues in his/her life will certainly ask, "What are you committed to? What is important to you? What do you believe?" and will help the individual sort out his/her beliefs. The integration of personhood and health, a goal of the Wholistic Health Center, is seen as an inherently religious concept of life.

Being grounded deeply in faith, the pastoral counselors can listen for expressions reflecting the strength of the human spirit. The pastoral counselors know that faith is not just the right words, but a stance from which one views life and out of which one makes decisions. The pastoral counselors seek to promote the well-being (*shalom*) of a strong human spirit.

The pastoral counselors are not "special ministers" working outside the church context. They are pastors called by a local church community. They involve themselves in the life of that worshipping community and gain personal support from it, as well as interpret the role of health in the ministry of the church to it. Most volunteers and support group programs utilized at the Wholistic Health Centers emerge from the context of the local churches.

The pastoral counselors, by their participation in the health team within the context of a family practice medical center, have learned to be more sensitive to medical issues and how they relate to social, emotional, and spiritual health. Although they refrain from giving medical advice, they do attend to issues such as weight, exercise, blood pressure, and current medications. They do carefully read the medical history and medical status reports as they involve themselves in a counseling relationship with a patient.

*WHY A PASTORAL COUNSELOR?*    Since the role of a pastoral counselor in health care is not as well understood or as universally accepted as that of the nurse and the physician, some amplification on the function of the pastoral counselor in the Wholistic Health Center setting might be helpful.

The pastoral counselor is an important member of the health care team because of the relationship between life stress and health, and the centrality of spiritual issues in the coping with this stress. At its most fundamental level, the handling of life stresses boils down to a series of spiritual questions that indicate a person's outlook on life.

> What is the aim of my life? (Meaning-Purpose-Goal)
> What beliefs and values guide me? (Faith)
> What do I choose to spend myself on? (Commitment)
> What am I willing to let go of? (Surrender)

Two examples can illustrate these ideas. A young man came to the Center with hypertension and backaches. He had been working 70 hours per week. He hoped to get a raise so his family could live better. He had tremendous drive to succeed and always seemed to be in a hurry.

His physical problems were real (hypertension and backaches); his spiritual problems were also real. We asked him:

> "My friend, where are you going so fast? And why?" (Meaning)
> "What do you believe? Are you the center of the universe or is there something, Someone, beyond you?" (Faith)
> "How are you spending your time and energy? Are you spending it on what you really want to commit yourself and life to?" (Commitment)

"Can you surrender, let go of some control, acknowledge that life is a terminal illness?" (Surrender)

"You are mortal. Can you *trust* enough in God in the
fact that others can love, accept, forgive you, even
if you're not perfect?" (Surrender)

Yes, he could, and did. He found that there is another
way of looking at life, and he began to deal with his disease
and stress.

A woman came to the Center with nagging headaches,
recent weight gain, and a feeling of depression. She recently had experienced great changes in her life. She had
stopped working outside the home, two close friends had
moved away, and the children had grown up and left home.
We reflected with her:

"My friend, it looks like you've shut yourself off from
other people. It sounds like you're grieving over the
loss of life as you had it 6 months ago, and you can't
seem to say good-bye to the past and reinvest yourself in the present." (Meaning)

"Can we look for your values? What's important to
you?" (Faith)

"Can we together search out the commitments you
wish to make?" (Commitment)

"Can you find a renewed sense of hope and meaning?" (Surrender)

"Can you be freed from the feeling of being trapped?"
(Surrender)

Yes, she could, and did. She found ways of restoring
meaning and commitment in her life by reinvesting herself
in others. The stress-related backaches and headaches
cleared up in the process.

People's stress level, and ultimately their health, is partly determined by their answers to spiritual questions.

In listening to and responding (hopefully creatively) to the wide range of stresses and personal disease experienced by people, the Wholistic Health Center's counselor is both pastor and health care provider.

In attempting to accept, encourage, and goad (kick) people into taking care of themselves, in offering a disquieting question, in struggling with people looking for meaning who need to make some commitments, who need to both take control of their lives and surrender some things that are beyond their control, in attempting to offer love, forgiveness, and a quiet word of hope, and in helping people to accept the fact that it's okay that they're not perfect, the Wholistic Health Center's pastoral counselor is both pastor and health care provider.

In being a member of a team of people with a variety of helping skills, all primarily interested in developing a sense of wholeness, increasing the quality of life, and promoting the fullness of health among those who come to the Wholistic Health Center, the Wholistic Health Center's pastoral counselor is both pastor and health care provider.

## The Role of Volunteers

Forty years ago, when volunteers approached hospitals wanting to be useful and helpful in patient care, hospital administrators had no idea what to do with them. There were no precedents for people who weren't paid to become a part of the staff. Volunteer programs were revolutionary. Today most hospitals would have to increase significantly their already exorbitant daily bed rate if the volunteers were not available.

Dr. Russell Mawby, President of the Kellogg Foundation, believes that throughout the history of America the spirit of volunteerism has been behind a great many significant improvements in personal services (Mawby, 1976). Volunteers have often been utilized to perform "human services" that would not "pay for themselves." Today most outpatient medical clinics would have no idea what to do if some volunteers suddenly appeared at the door wanting to help. It's possible that 30 years from now we will look back and say, "How did we ever get along without the help of faithful volunteers?"

The Wholistic Health Center is based on the principle of volunteerism. Secretary-receptionists, nurses, pastoral counselors, patients helping other patients, and "special friends" are all volunteers involved in the program of the Wholistic Health Center. How else could we spend the kind of time we do without doubling our fees? The churches of our country have always been a source of willing and able people wanting to help with significant causes. Sometimes they have been condescendingly labeled "do gooders." The fact is that there's a wealth of talent and human energy waiting to be tapped by the ambulatory health care system of America. In the Wholistic Health Center we are learning to take seriously the fact that pay is not a prerequisite for being helpful to another person in need.

The Wholistic Health Centers utilize the services of persons in professional roles who simply are not paid money. No volunteers are free; they must receive satisfaction or education for their time, or they will not stay involved. In addition, the Wholistic Health Centers utilize a number of laypersons who have been patients of the Center to help persons with difficulties similar to those they have experienced. Other volunteers help with accounting, business management, architectural planning, interior design, physical repairs, and the like. As the Wholistic Health Centers have grown, the involvement of volunteers has increased, although specific jobs have changed noticeably. Whereas earlier efforts concentrated on physical improvements, today there's room for volunteers in various steps of the patient care system.

A number of issues have arisen and been dealt with concerning volunteers in our medical facility. First, we have had to work out definite levels of "Clearance" for access to records. We take the confidentiality of patient records very seriously. Obviously, for a clinic located in a church, "security" of information is a paramount consideration. The general rule is that the right to information on the "problem" of the patient is directly related to the level of responsibility for the care of that patient. The receptionist needs to know little about the personal health problem. The nurse needs to know as much as possible. Neither need to know anything about patients other than those whom they are directly servicing with care.

Second, a specific "contract" is worked out with each volunteer. How long will you be with us? What will you do? Here's what you can expect over that time from us. "We'll evaluate our mutual contract together on __(date)__." Those are the considerations included in our mutual understanding.

Third, the orientation and training of the volunteers is a process that must be taken seriously, especially within the teamwork approach. People need to know each other in order to be able to work together effectively. They need to know the specific job they are asked to do, and they need to know what the Wholistic Health Center is all about.

With the volunteer pastoral counselors we have learned that we need to require a long-term commitment of 9 months to 1 year. The pastor can work for as few as 3 to 4 hours a week, but he/she must be available over a long period of time in order to justify the training investment and the assigning of counselees, who may need help for an undetermined length of time. Since there is so much to learn with the medical and teamwork emphases, only those pastors who are already skilled counselors can really benefit from participation as volunteers. The Wholistic Health Center is no place to learn elementary counseling skills.

## Professional Functions within the Initial Health Planning Conference

Since the uniqueness of the teamwork approach is most clearly demonstrated in the Initial Health Planning Conference, we will examine in more detail the way each staff person functions in facilitating the effective management of that Conference (Peterson et al., 1976). It is important to include a description of the patients' responsibilities as well, since the patients are considered full members of the team.

In a Health Planning Conference where three different professional people work together as a team, it is not enough to assume that the secretary, nurse, physician, and pastoral counselor have mutually exclusive roles that they all understand. Instead of merely enacting the usual professional roles, the staff members become managers of a number of processes that are going on simultaneously. The effectiveness of the Planning Conference depends on the successful management of these processes: (1) the patients' process of engagement; (2) the secretary's process of entry and exit; (3) the nurse's process of advocacy; (4) the physician's process of physical assessment; and (5) the counselor's process of life-position assessment. These processes take place in parallel during patients' first visits.

Staff members do not ask themselves, "Am I in my role?"; instead they ask themselves, "Is the process for which I am responsible being facilitated effectively?"

### The Patients' Process of Engagement

The patients' process of engagement begins with the first phone call to the Center, or possibly even earlier, when they hear about the Center from someone else. The process begins with people's decision to come to us at a time when they still probably know very little about us. The engagement process focuses patients' attention not only on the question of, "What is wrong with me?", but also on questions such as, "What kind of a place is this? What kind of people will see me? What will they ask me? Can these people be trusted? Is all of our conversation in confidence? Why do I need all of these people to sit down with me?"

An important aspect of the patients' process is the recognition that defining and treating their problem is only a part of their progress toward health. People must become actively engaged in the process of taking care of themselves as well. They must, in the process of engagement, develop a sense of confidence in themselves and in the staff of the Center. Patients need to hear that their decisions are supported, affirmed, and respected. They must cultivate a sense of accountability to themselves. They need to understand that when a plan is developed, the team at the Center will support them with assistance, but that they alone can be accountable for carrying out the plan.

The process of engagement must foster the feeling for patients that they are trusted to take care of themselves and are expected to do so, and that these expectations are realistic. It is never acceptable at the Wholistic Health Center for people to become merely "passive good patients." The outcome of the process must be that patients are engaged in the active venture of taking care of themselves.

*The Secretary's Process of Entry and Exit*

The secretary is responsible for the smooth operation of the Center on a daily basis. She/he supervises clerical and receptionist volunteers, prepares and records billings and payments, answers the phone, keeps appointment schedules, and performs (or finds volunteers to assist with) tasks that are deemed necessary by the treatment team. She/he explains over the phone what the Wholistic Health Center is all about and describes the Initial Health Planning Conference. If patients understand the purpose of the Conference and are sold on the concept, they are more likely to participate in a frame of mind that will allow them the maximum benefit.

After the Conference, the secretary and receptionists often gather valuable feedback about the satisfaction of patients with the Conference and their understanding of the plan that was developed. The secretary makes sure that patients experience as smooth an entry and exit as possible.

The secretary and receptionists (usually volunteers) have a significant effect on the outcome of the Initial Health Planning Conference. Their importance as part of the health care team should not be minimized.

*The Nurse's Process of Advocacy*

In the Initial Health Planning Conference the nurse manages the development of an advocacy relationship with patients, being sure that people understand what we do, what we don't do, and that we do intend to listen carefully to them. Following the Conference, the nurse ensures that patients understand the plans that were developed and that they know what will be expected of them.

The nurse is the first person who touches patients, emotionally and physically. She/he establishes a rapport and a sense of trust that she/he and the patient share as they enter the Planning Conference together.

Advocacy also includes the nurse's responsibility to make sure that patients' concerns are heard. She/he does this by eliciting comments from patients if they seem hesitant to share something with the staff that they previously shared with her/him, and by being open to patients' comments about their feelings about being at the Center.

The nurse usually remains relatively quiet during the Conference. If patients are dissatisfied with the Conference, the nurse remains a safe person with whom they can share their complaints.

## The Physician's Process of Physical Assessment

In the Planning Conference the physician manages the process of physical assessment from a Wholistic perspective, listening for nonmedical concerns as well as physical symptoms. The physician often needs to know what people's previous experience with physicians has been in order to assess their attitudes toward health care providers. The physician explores the possible relationships between physical symptoms and people's style of life and, in addition, attempts to sense which treatment alternatives patients will be most likely to follow. Of course, in the cases of obvious physical disease, the physician does recommend very specific treatments.

As the manager of a process instead of an interrogator, the physician may choose to sit and listen while another member of the team explores physical problems. Often the physician gains considerable additional insight into people's physical health as well as their attitudes by listening as they talk with another team member. This process also allows the physician more time to consider a diagnosis.

In the Initial Health Planning Conference, the physician is allowed to practice the diagnostic skills of medicine without being expected to handle problems inappropriate for medical care. The presence of two other professionals means that the doctor can probe, explore, and confront patients in an atmosphere of trust and respect. It is almost paradoxical that effective scientific medicine may be most possible in the context of a wholistic, interdisciplinary practice.

## The Pastoral Counselor's Process of Life-Position Assessment

In the Initial Health Planning Conference, the pastoral counselor manages the process of life-position assessment. The counselor needs to know what is happening in people's lives, how they feel about themselves, how they see their faith, and who the significant other people are in their lives at the moment.

In order to assess people's life-position, the pastoral counselor evaluates the amount of change they have recently experienced in their lives and tries to sense whether they are in a state of crisis, transition, or stability. Utilizing this assessment, the pastoral counselor can be very helpful in putting together a realistic plan for people. Persons in crisis, for example, are not ready to tackle long-term plans designed to help them stop smoking or lose weight. People in crisis need to know how to survive. Persons in transition need to be able to grieve and move on in order to meet new challenges. People in a relatively stable life situation are much more ready to engage in long-term treatment, to think about developing a healthy life-style, and to take care of themselves over a long period of time. Life-position assessment also includes questions about the person's faith in terms of what they believe about themselves and about the world, and an assessment of what they feel needs to happen in their lives.

Essentially, the counselor seeks to ascertain the kinds of needs that have led persons to come to the Center, the level of their motivation to change, and the behavior patterns they want to change in the near future.

*Coordinating the Processes*

Obviously the process of engagement, entry and exit, advocacy, physical assessment, and life-position assessment overlap. Staff members at the Center learn from each other. The counselor, over a period of time watching the physician, learns the kinds of questions to ask in relation to physical symptoms. The physician and the nurse learn from the counselor some skills in exploring and assessing people's life-position. All staff members learn from the secretary some skills in time management. From the patients of the Center we are continually learning better ways of engaging people to care for themselves. Each specific process, however, is still managed by the appropriate staff member who is responsible for its completion.

Parallel process also requires that the patients be involved as participants. The members of the staff cannot make decisions for patients. Patients must ultimately make and own the decisions as part of their own process of engagement.

## THE NEED FOR FLEXIBILITY

The teamwork approach is difficult for the staff at times because of the flexibility demanded. During the Initial Health Planning Conference, for instance, we almost never know where we're headed or the problems patients will bring up. We must be honest when we don't know something. We need faith in the process, love for each other, and confidence in ourselves in order to make ourselves maximally available to patients, to follow the direction the Conference takes, and to respond in a way that will ultimately be helpful.

At times, staff members may be called on to do things that their professional colleagues in other settings would see as inappropriate or out of line. That kind of flexibility, however, is required for wholistic health care to occur effectively. In a recent team study, flexibility was the primary quality named by the staff as being necessary for joining the team at the Wholistic Health Center.

Each staff person is responsible for bringing his/her specific area of expertise to bear on the problems of patients. Physicians at the Wholistic Health Center are not expected to be counselors, nor are counselors expected to handle medical diagnosis and treatment.

However, the staff is flexible and not possessive when

a staff member is able to help with problems normally considered to be in another's "professional territory." The consistent goal is that all of the needs be managed effectively so that patients feel cared about and encouraged to make important decisions about their own health.

For participation in this kind of teamwork, each of the professional people must be highly competent and have sufficient self-confidence to share their responsibilities with others. It is probable that Wholistic Health Centers require staff people who are more competent professionally and more self-confident about their own professional and personal identity than would be required in other kinds of health care settings.

## SUMMARY

Within the context of the Wholistic Health Centers the distinct professional expertise of each staff member is utilized, while at the same time allowing each to invest a wide variety of personal sensitivities and skills in the creation of a caring relationship with patients. The unique blend of professional and personal expertise embodied within each Wholistic Health Center team fosters an atmosphere of creativity in encounters with patients, and increases the likelihood that patients will experience a positive response to the variety of problems for which they seek help.

*Chapter 9*

# PRIMARY MODALITIES OF CARE IN THE WHOLISTIC HEALTH CENTER

The philosophy of the Wholistic Health Center dictates that the staff responds to a variety of needs. Our approach also frees the staff to formulate creative, unexpected, treatment plans together with the patient.

Many of those who have commented on the state of primary health care have called for the coordination of health services and the broadening of the services rendered. If lack of a babysitter keeps a mother from receiving health care for herself, then some babysitting help must be found before she will avail herself of the services. Providing transportation, being open at convenient hours, meeting the patient on his/her "home ground," and recruiting volunteers to assist with these needs are all activities in which the Wholistic Health Center staff has engaged.

The primary modalities of care utilized in the Wholistic Health Centers generally fall into two areas: crisis care for sickness and educational care to prevent illness. The crisis care is usually direct medical or counseling service.

The preventive-educational care consists of one-to-one teaching and health education seminars for larger groups of people. In a sense, everything we do has an intended educational component, since we're constantly attempting, even in crisis care, to help people to take a more wholistic view of their health and assume greater personal responsibility for maintaining it themselves.

Figure 9.1 indicates the types of services rendered at the Wholistic Health Center and provides a basic outline of the material in this chapter.

## CRISIS CARE

Crisis care for acute disease is the *sine qua non* of any health provider's work. In the case of the Wholistic Health Centers, crisis care can either be emergency medical care for acute illness or supportive counseling care for traumatic social or emotional upheaval.

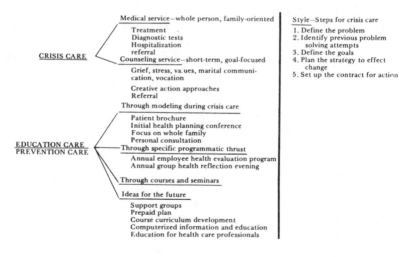

**Figure 9.1   Modalities of Care**

*MEDICAL SERVICE.*    Medical care services are offered in a manner similar to any other family practice clinic, with the exception of tests and procedures that need more sophisticated equipment than is available in the Center. For these procedures, patients are referred to a hospital laboratory, which has agreed to handle all our speciality tests, or a local private laboratory. In addition to the technical medical care, the physician spends a reasonable amount of time with each patient, listening, explaining procedures, and giving information.

Some normal medical procedures are carried out with a different emphasis because of our wholistic and family-focused philosophy. For example, at times the whole family is encouraged to have a health checkup and planning conference together. Husbands are encouraged to accompany their wives for O.B.-Gyn. concerns. Our philosophy challenges us to look continually for more humanistic ways to deliver medical technology.

*COUNSELING SERVICE.*    Counseling services include individual, marital, family, and group contexts, depending on the needs of the patient (s) and the theoretical base and inclination of the particular counselor. Most counseling is short-term and goal-focused. Themes we deal with most often are transition and grief, managing stress, clarifying values, personal-emotional issues, spiritual faith, marital and family communication, and vocational concerns.

## General Approach to Crisis Care

The uniqueness of our care lies not so much in the individual activities of counseling or medical care, but in the emphases that flow from the wholistic approach. The wholistic philosophy, offered by an interdisciplinary team of professionals, almost "forces" people to take a look at the whole picture of their health. We ask them about all aspects of life and health, and are certain to bring up aspects of life that are noticeably not mentioned by the patient.

This focus is the source of the unusual creativity and variety found in the treatment approaches we have employed. Almost no activity is "out of bounds" or too far-fetched. Any activity can be potentially helpful, and all sides of life (physical, emotional, social, spiritual) are searched for creative possibilities for treatment.

If a husband and wife fight every Thursday night when the husband flies home from his regular out-of-town work-week, we may meet him at the airport and try to work through some of the "reentry issues." We'll talk over a cup of coffee at a restaurant. We've asked people to walk around the block once before responding in a marital fight. We've asked them to listen to organ music, to make a phone call once a day to someone in need, to paint signs for the Center, and so on. We'll set up a "contract" with people to do almost anything that might work.

We get people to read books; we've found them places to volunteer; and we've sent them to Parent Effectiveness Training classes, to health spas, to Marriage Encounter weekends, and to Gestalt workshops. We've told them to go fishing, or "go fly a kite" (perhaps sometimes this is intended mainly to improve our own health and manage our own stress!). We've put people in touch with groups of parents of exceptional children, groups for parents who have lost a child, emotional health support groups, "koinonia" support and sharing groups structured by the Christian Laymen of Chicago, cancer patients' support groups, weight control groups, and the like.

Our goal in all these activities is to do anything possible to get the patients back in touch with their own resources and in touch with the support of others around them who can help by understanding and caring.

Some patients are referred to other agencies or professionals for part of their health care, either medical or counseling. The Wholistic Health Center staff therefore serves as coordinators. This is a service we take seriously as a viable and essential treatment modality.

*The Process Steps in Crisis Care*

The style of our care for both medical and nonmedical problems usually follows a common process of defining the problem, setting the goals, and formulating a strategy for reaching those goals. This process starts with, but is not isolated to, the Initial Health Planning Conference.

We consistently ask ourselves and our patients three questions that help to clarify what the patient wants and how we can help.

> *What is your problem?* (We try to get people to be very specific in spelling out the needs they feel.)
> *Why did you come here to this Center now?* (What forced you to make the decision to get help—and why did you come to us?)
> *What do you expect from us?*

We attempt to raise these and similar questions not only on the initial visit, but as treatment continues in order for both the patient and provider to take stock of where they're at and where they're headed.

Let's look at the process embodied in our style of crisis care and isolate the steps we usually follow.

*1. DEFINING THE PROBLEM.*    The patient has a problem, a concern for which the patient needs our expertise. Often the patient has a very clear idea of what the problem is and exactly what treatment is needed. For example, a woman who feels "uptight" and wants a prescription for "something I can take for my nerves" is describing to us both her diagnosis and her treatment plan.

The trick for us often is the necessity to redefine the

problem. We must broaden the patient's focus and take a look at the whole life. Perhaps then we'll find the real cause behind the symptoms and can identify the strengths and resources on which the individual can draw in handling the problem. We soon discover that the woman who feels "uptight" is really grieving over the loss of identity she has felt since her children all left home and she has no one to care for who needs her attention. The problem is then redefined, and a wide range of solutions are available—solutions that are more creative than a lifetime prescription for Valium three times daily. Perhaps her desire and ability to care for others is needed somewhere in her community and she can turn her strength into a treatment plan for healing her "nerves" as well as helping others.

Often the treatment becomes obvious once the problem is defined accurately.

*2. IDENTIFYING THE PROBLEM SOLVING THAT HAS GONE ON ALREADY.* The question we ask is, "What have you tried so far? Why hasn't it been successful?" People have always tried to handle problems themselves. They may have tried more rest, getting together with friends, drinking, working harder, over-the-counter remedies, and the like. Invariably, when they come for professional care, it's because all the attempts they have made at solving the problem have failed and they have run out of ideas. Sometimes the attempts to solve one problem have caused a new problem. For example, excessive eating, drinking, or working to deaden painful feelings often cause undesirable side effects. We listen to what people have already tried. Most of the time people have tried many variations on a similar theme and have not been terribly creative about dreaming up totally new problem-solving attempts. A housewife with small children may not need a different tranquilizer (more of the same); instead, she may need to get out of the house, away from her children 3 or 4 hours a week.

*3. DEFINITION OF THE GOALS.*       The simple question that gets at the definition of goals is, "What do you want?" Most often people will answer this question in general terms like, "I want to be happy." It's our job to help them define their wants in specific terms. We may ask, "What would make you happy?" The answers "a good marriage," "to get rid of my headaches," "to take a vacation," may lead to specific goals that can be clarified and worked toward. It's our job to help the individual define goals that are possible. The goal "I want my husband back from the dead" is a difficult one for which to plan treatment. The goal "I want to learn to live without him" is more possible.

Sometimes people have spent so much time complaining about their problems and all the terrible things that have happened to them that they don't really know what they want. Behind every complaint is a need. As long as the complaining continues, energy is generally not being spent in the search for a solution. If people have been stuck in complaining, the question "What do you want?" may prove helpful to shock them into taking some action on their own behalf and stopping the endless game of repeating "Ain't it awful" to everyone who will listen.

*4. PLANNING STRATEGY TO EFFECT THE DESIRED CHANGE.*       After (re-)defining the problem, finding what's been tried before, and establishing the goals, we're ready to start looking for some new ways of moving toward the goal and solving the problems; we're ready to formulate a treatment plan.

Our expertise and task is to help people imagine another way different from those they have tried before. Frequently we find that the "other way" comes naturally out of either the redefinition of the problem or establishment of the goals. Once these first two tasks are accomplished, the strategy for making the change is often obvious. To get at this we usually ask, "Given this awful situation you're in, how could you take care of yourself and begin to get what you want?" Very likely patients will come up with ideas they had not considered before in answer to this question.

At times, we've found that a careful analysis of a person's strengths will indicate possible untapped resources that can assist them in the change process. We bring all the dimensions of the whole person into play when attempting to dream up treatment ideas that may be effective. The combination and variety of ideas that come out of this search are enormous.

*5. SETTING THE CONTRACT.*      Finally, we and the patient together settle on a plan of action based on the creative ideas that have been generated in Step 4. The patient and the treatment team must select one or a number of plans that will be enacted. Which idea looks like it might help? Which is the patient ready to try? Before closing a session, everyone needs to be clear on what is to be tried and *how* we can evaluate whether it's successful or not. The results —whether the planned treatment works or not—will feed back into the next session as material for helping to redefine the problem, establish goals, and so forth, beginning the sorting process all over again.

### Summary of the Process

In crisis care our goal is, as quickly as possible, to get people moving and caring for themselves again. We try to help them to get information, visualize alternative solutions, and formulate action experiences that they need to carry out in order to regain control of their lives and their health. Thus, we tend to be short-term, action-oriented instead of long-term, analysis-insight oriented in our treatments.

We believe people know where they want to go and that they have the right, responsibility, and ability to decide in which direction they will go and the number of steps they will take. For people to get maximum benefit from the helping process we employ, they must be willing to take control of themselves again. They may feel out of control, but they must be willing to act on their own behalf, no matter how they feel. Persons who won't exercise self-control, diminish our ability to be helpful to them.

*Issues in Crisis Care*

Three additional issues related to our patient care treatment style deserve mention.

*WHO GETS COUNSELING?*    Do we seduce people into counseling? The answer is "No." It is true that we let people know that counseling is available at the Center, but we rarely suggest to people who come strictly for medical care that they should engage in counseling. When people come for sore throats or warts, the sore throats and warts are treated medically. We do not ask people for information that they aren't comfortable telling us. We do not try to "create problems" in areas of their lives for which patients are not asking for help. Patients are not required to show us their Personal Health Inventory unless they choose to do so.

We do attempt, however, to influence how people look at their health and how they deal with their health problems. When health problems occur, we offer them the opportunity to go through the process of sorting out their health problems and behaviors and finding a better way to care for themselves. Some accept the offer; others do not. Each patient is always in charge of that decision.

*HOW DO YOU OFFER THE SPIRITUAL CARE?*    Do we push religion? The answer is "No." However, this is a question we wrestle with often. Just as feelings are often confusing and have to be talked through with a good listener in order to be understood, so also spiritual and faith-related beliefs are often confusing and need to be talked through and reflected clearly by another person before an individual is able to clarify them for himself/herself. Just as we don't tell people how to feel, we also don't tell them what to believe.

We try to find out as much about patients' spiritual lives as we do about their physical condition, social situation, and emotional well-being. Questions and comments such as the following often open the door.

1.  "Do you consider yourself a religious person?"
2.  "What part does God play in your life?"
3.  "Sounds like you're in a religious dilemma."

We try to let our patients know that the Wholistic Health Center is a place where they can explore questions of faith because we're willing to take the risks with them.

One staff memo, however, raises clearly the dilemma we face.

> "Sometimes we have had difficulty approaching or responding to religious or spiritual questions raised by our patients —for example:
>
>   Why does God let this happen?
>   What good does it do to believe?
>   I have given my life to Jesus; what more can I do?
>
> Much of our difficulty probably comes from our expectations of ourselves to have the answers to these unanswerable questions. Nevertheless, I think that if we do not encourage exploration of religious questions and mutually explore our patients' faith, we may be engaged in a form of malpractice of wholistic health care. Let's keep this issue alive among ourselves.

Wholistic Health Centers have grown out of a conviction that one's faith and outlook on life are integral to the health and healing of the body. If health care fails to deal with the spiritual dimension, the patient is not being treated as a whole person. We believe that most medical facilities avoid the religious dimension as if it played no role in health care.

A person's value system and faith must be a part of the staff's concern. However, the staff must find their way between no mention whatsoever of the spiritual aspect of life on the one hand, and hitting the patient with questions such as "Are you saved?" on the other.

One of the considerations seems to be that there are times when people are receptive to spiritual reflection; at other times, they simply are not. There are a few times when the spiritual barges in on our lives and we are ready to deal with it; at other times, we are not ready and don't sense the need at all.

The question for us seems to be finding a way of dealing with the spiritual and meeting patients' needs, offering to reflect with them about spiritual concerns without pushing them to deal with issues for which they do not desire our help.

*HOW DO YOU BREAK DOWN ISOLATION OF PEOPLE?*    Isn't loneliness the cause of much disease? We believe it is. One of the biggest health problems we face is the sense of isolation among people. Isolation can be the result of a problem (someone who died, or a person too sick to be socially active). Isolation is also the cause of new problems. The need to "go it alone," especially when hurting, cuts people off from a great deal of support and creative ideas for changing the problem. One of the great tragedies of the health care system is that it has, for the most part, opted to treat people alone—one by one. People come in the door, wait silently, see the physician, counselor, minister, or nurse, and go back home, once again isolated with their problem.

As part of our treatment approach, we have tried to foster the image of the Wholistic Health Center as more than a professional crisis care center. We try to communicate that "When you're a patient here, you're a member." The Wholistic Health Center is a place where people can get involved, a place to belong. We try to foster friendships between patients and offer educational support groups for those who feel the need. Many patients join the continually growing cadre of volunteers who invest time and expertise in a wide range of activities related to the Centers.

## PREVENTION AND HEALTH EDUCATION

The need for health education and prevention programs designed to help people change illness-producing behaviors is enormous. However, most health care is focused on episodic crises, not on long-term prevention. Why? It is both because crises, by their very nature, demand immediate attention and because it is difficult to make health education programs financially self-supporting.

In Wholistic Health Centers, we are serious about health education, and we are managing to sell preventive services. We certainly aren't doing as much education as we are crisis care and we, too, see the tempting truth that we could become self-supporting faster by focusing on crisis care than by "fooling with" preventive and educational services. But we haven't given in to the pressures. Education is still a major part of what we do. We presently fall far short of our vision of what's possible in education and prevention. When seen in the context of what isn't happening in the rest of the country, however, we have already been extremely successful.

### Patient Education as a Style of Care

Much of the prevention and education emphasis within the Wholistic Health Centers is based on the modeling and structuring of diagnosis and planning that occurs within the Health Planning Conference. A major nonverbal and verbal message of this conference is, "You are responsible to care for your own health!" This in itself, if accepted by the patient, is a significant step toward patient education and, hopefully, behavior change.

*PATIENT EDUCATION THROUGH WRITTEN BROCHURE.*    We have experimented with written descriptions designed to teach patients how they can best help themselves. Excerpts from one such "brochure" we have used are included below.

### ON BEING A GOOD PATIENT AT THE WHOLISTIC HEALTH CENTER
How You Can Help Us Help You

If you want to get the best of what we can give, you'll have to be active on your own behalf.

*What can you expect when you come to us for health care?*

You can expect that we will assume that you have resources with which to manage your life, but are presently having difficulty sorting them out and utilitizing them.

We will further assume that you ultimately wish to maintain the responsibility for yourself and your own road back to health.

You can expect that we will resist any attempt by you to make the problem or solution external to yourself.

We will listen as intently as possible in the attempt to understand your concerns, and with the hope that we might reflect to you blind spots and inconsistent patterns of which you are not aware.

We will attempt to recognize and accept feelings of unworthiness (guilt) expressed about yourself, and to communicate to you that these also can be accepted by you.

We will attempt to help you regain a sense of hope, for as you begin to expect the movement toward health, you will help make it occur.

*The process of asking for help means that you've already done a lot of work and decision making before you made the appointment.*

We're pleased you've already done a lot of work on your own ... we want to take that seriously ... your ideas are

important, we want to hear your thoughts . . . and we'll, of course, share ours. We're pleased now that you've come, we ask you to keep on working—sorting out yourself.
We need you to be active to help us know how to help in the best way we can . . . help you get what you want for yourself and your health.
We need you to be part of the team in our healing partnership. How can we go about this process together?
*Every attempt at health care is based on a relationship.*
Relationships don't thrive on guessing each other's needs. If we try to read your mind, guess what you want, we might hit it right a few times, but we will also miss, and you'll feel hurt.
If you try to read our minds and guess what we want you might be right some of the time, but you'll also be wrong some . . . and you won't get the purpose of your visit accomplished.
We—you and we—need to talk about what we want from each other. Neither of us can guess . . . or read the other's mind. Because relationships thrive on open discussion of what each person needs.

Our mutual relationship of helping is based not only on caring for each other during the time we are together, but also on some expertise which we share with each other.
Your expertise is you—your pain, fear, life-style, goals, willingness to work.
Our expertise is ourselves—our training and experience—which give us some special ability in assisting with health problems whether physical or "human spirit."
We need to be able to share our expertise together as we make plans for improving your health, and then begin to carry them out.

Through this kind of written challenge to patients, we are doing patient education. We are teaching people that it is important for them to take care of themselves responsibly and participate fully in the healing process. We are attempting to change attitudes of passive dependency to new attitudes of independence and personal responsibility. We are restructuring our relationships with patients so that healing has a better chance of taking place in our encounters with them.

*PATIENT EDUCATION THROUGH THE HEALTH PLANNING CONFERENCE.*
The Health Planning Conference serves as a mechanism that we can use for confronting people with negative, recurring, episodic, crisis care patterns as we see them develop. When, over a period of months, we notice that an individual has utilized our crisis care services on a fairly rhythmic, patterned basis, we can initiate a health planning and consultation conference in which we essentially say, "We've seen a pattern and want to offer you help in dealing with the pattern instead of just patching you up all the time." In this case we, as a team, sit with patients and confront them with what we see; we offer to look for ways to prevent regular recurrence of the crises. Our way of making such a confrontation palatable is the communication of the message, "If you want to be smart and want to get the maximum benefit from the service we have to offer, then you'll look for a way to change some of your behavior patterns and prevent the onset of illness."

*PREVENTION THROUGH VIEWING TOTAL LIFE AND FAMILY CONTEXT.*
Within the Wholistic Health Center, as a family medical center, we have easy entry into viewing the marital relationship and the family as a system. The Center setup, with the medical focus, provides a vehicle for offering counseling to people who would not otherwise seek it directly. The Initial Health Planning conference and the Annual Health Planning Conference provide excellent opportunities for reflection and assessment.

People go to a physician when they are physically ill, expecting a child, reaching a change of life, and at many other developmental stages. As part of a family practice medical care facility, staff members are able to have therapeutic contact with individuals and families over the breadth of their life span and developmental stages. As the

Center staff sees itself with the task of influencing people in all dimensions of life toward health, including marital health, it is able to offer prevention and enrichment within family relationships instead of just first aid.

We are working on the plans for a yearly whole health checkup for the entire family. This will include a medical examination and planning conference for each individual family member, and a joint reflection and planning meeting focused on family communication for the entire family together. Perhaps we will also use a short audiovisual program on family interaction that the family could view and discuss among themselves.

*PATIENT EDUCATION THROUGH PERSONAL CONSULTATION.*    Informal and individualized education is carried out in both counseling and medical services. The most common forms are teaching the grief process, developing an exercise program, relaxation training, diet and nutrition education, assistance in designing individualized weight control programs, and information on managing a variety of chronic diseases.

Although our physicians patiently spend a great deal of time teaching about health issues and disease management, most of the one-to-one educational counseling is done by nurses. Each nurse tends to focus on one or two specific education areas at which she/he becomes expert.

In all of these efforts emphasis is placed on the formulation of specific behavioral contracts designed to fit the individual patient's preferences and needs. Some people need to check in with us each week for support. Others take the plan and work with it by themselves for a month or more before checking back with us.

*Specific Health Care Preventive Programs*

Two specific programs that offer health planning and prevention as a major thrust have been integrated into the regular health care services of the Center. These are the Annual Employee Health Evaluation Program for Business Owners and the Annual Group Health Reflection Evening for patients.

*THE ANNUAL EMPLOYEE HEALTH EVALUATION PROGRAM FOR BUSINESS OWNERS.* The program is based on the assumption that healthy, well-motivated people who care about themselves are the core of a productive, creative business enterprise. Employee annual health evaluations with Wholistic Health Centers are intended to engage the employees in the process of becoming healthy, whole people who are responsible for themselves. This program is designed to replace the annual physical examination for employees offered by many companies.

The Employee Health Evaluation program screens for early detection of illness such as heart disease and cancer as well as health-threatening stresses of employment or life changes. The evaluation focuses time and attention on the greatest threats to health instead of on expensive, unnecessary tests and procedures. In addition, the evaluation supports employees' decisions to care for themselves by, for example, developing an exercise plan, controlling alcohol and drug intake, or engaging in problem solving with a spouse.

The evaluation may include an optional, on-site visit by a member of the Wholistic Health Center staff who is experienced in occupational and environmental stress. The visit consists of brief interviews with employees, a study of the environment, and a report to management with recommendations on stress control for the business as a whole.

The Annual Health Evaluation is a two-stage process during the first year with a more simplified process in following years. When an employee comes the first year, he/she is engaged in an Initial Planning Conference in which the clinic is described, any concerns about health are discussed, and necessary laboratory work is determined. In this conference, the employee is treated as a mutual participant in the plan, recognizing that he/she makes the important decisions about personal health care. Between the Initial Health Planning Conference and the physical examination, the employee visits a convenient laboratory and has the tests done; results are sent to the clinic in preparation for the return visit. The employee also fills out a health history questionnaire that is brought along when he/she returns.

The return visit (1-2 weeks later) consists of a physical examination, a review of the laboratory work, and a debriefing conference where the results of the evaluation are summarized and recommendations are mutually discussed. If the employee requests it, we send his/her physician a copy of the evaluation results. Normally, no information from the evaluation is shared with the employer other than the fact that the employee did come for the evaluation.

For evaluations in following years, the employee talks with the clinic physician by telephone to arrange for necessary laboratory work and comes in only for the physical examination and debriefing conference. Figure 9.2 illustrates the process for the initial year.

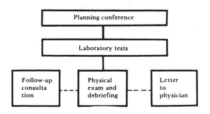

**Figure 9.2**

*ANNUAL GROUP HEALTH REFLECTION EVENING.*    We have designed a 2-hour program intended to engage patients in a seminar-type self-assessment of their health and analysis of their health behavior on a yearly basis. Patients audit their records, participate in a variety of reflection goal-setting and sharing exercises, and at the end of the evening, record the results of their evening's work in their chart.

Advantages of this group planning conference over the individual conferences are the cost effectiveness in terms of staff time and the support that develops among clinic patients as a result of the group sharing process. Patients see others working on health behavior problems similar to their own. Some patients, threatened by the individual conference, find it possible to attend the group conference.

## Courses and Seminars

Formal educational/preventive programs have included seminar series on the creative management of stress, empathy training, weight control workshops, and stop smoking clinics. These courses have become the "bread and butter" of the health education efforts to this point. For the most part, they have been oversubscribed each time they have been taught.

Recently, we have experimented with teaching approximately 20 new courses on health-related topics, such as, The Psychology of Women, Taking Care of Yourself, and Communication Skills. Some of these new courses will undoubtedly develop momentum and be included as part of the "regular fare" offered to our patients and the community.

In addition to serving a need for health education within our general communities, the seminars also serve as major segments of the treatment plans developed for many patients. A patient having trouble managing stress in his/her life could either "purchase" six counseling sessions at $30 per hour ($180) or attend the six-session Creative Management of Stress course for $30. In many cases the benefits, although somewhat different, are approximately equal. Often persons attend the stress seminar, then set up one or two counseling sessions to work on individual items that still concern them. The seminars are thus an extremely efficient method of accomplishing* health education and life-style counseling for specific life problem issues.

An added advantage is that people experiencing similar life-health difficulties are put in touch with each other. They find they are not as alone as they thought, and they are able to supply support for each other.

## The Future

In spite of our continual efforts and significant successes in focusing on prevention and health education, we have found over the past years that crisis care tasks have continually consumed the majority of our energy and attention.

We are presently wondering whether every Wholistic Health Center should include a fifth full-time professional staff person, a Human Health Development Specialist, whose sole responsibility would be to attend to and develop the preventive and educational portion of clinic services. By enlisting the support of numerous volunteers who would develop specific areas of expertise and teach a regular curriculum of courses, we feel certain that the educational arm of the Center could more than support the additional budget expenditure, and we would ensure constant attention to the extremely important aspects of education for health maintenance.

As the educational component of the Wholistic Health Centers develops in the future, we envision that it will include additional attention to several other innovative health care services.

We hope to create support and educational networks

among the handicapped, chronically ill, aged, and youth, and among persons with similar life-style problems. Some of this self-help network is already available through separate community groups. It would, however, be unique as far as we know for a primary care health center to coordinate and promote the development of such groups with health education and illness prevention as the goal.

The creation of mutual interest self-help groups among healthy persons within our community of patients would extend the scope of our services. These groups could be led by volunteers and would offer support—a chance for regular reflections on issues of health with like-minded persons. Persons could search their life-style for self-destructive patterns and find healthy alternatives through the exchange of ideas and the role models provided by each other.

We are experimenting with the development of a pre-payment crisis care plan that would offer a discount to persons who participate in a minimum number of health education units each year. This would be an incentive to persons not presently inclined to pay attention to their own prevention and health education needs. It would be intended to reverse the present negative reward payment system by offering crisis care at a lower rate to those who are actively engaged in the process of maintaining their health.

Course materials are currently in the planning stage in the areas of: (1) stress management, (2) chronic illness, (3) aging, (4) grief and loss management, (5) training of lay volunteers, (6) family life education, (7) the wholistic approach to health, (8) substance abuse, and (9) nutrition and diet education. Many materials are available that focus on information giving from the perspective of one professional discipline, but few are available that focus on behavioral change and personal decision making from the wholistic perspective.

We hope to perfect a method for diagnosing the patient's educational needs through an instrument designed to assess what a patient doesn't yet know that he/she needs to know, and then developing the programmed instruction techniques to furnish that knowledge.

We plan to develop continuing education programs for health care professionals that would, as part of its focus, create training and support groups among health care professionals. These continuing education opportunities would, like those for patient education, focus on attitude reassessment and behavior adjustment of faulty and unhealthy coping mechanisms commonly utilized by professionals. The twofold purpose of such an effort would be to (1) sensitize professionals to the wholistic needs of their patients, and (2) offer the professionals a rare opportunity to examine their own personal health issues and life-style.

## SUMMARY

Our treatment modalities for both crisis care and preventive health education are based on principles that will most likely remain constant in our future. The specific methodologies employed, however, are in a constant state of flux as we together create and test out additional methods for promoting a higher, more integrated level of health among those who seek our care.

*Chapter 10*

# THE PLACE OF THE WHOLISTIC
# HEALTH CENTER IN THE
# AMERICAN SYSTEM

No individual health care agency can offer satisfactory health care if it is isolated from other components of the health care structure. Many cults develop that offer the layperson some special "answers" to their health problems. Presently, many of those involved with these narrow, extreme approaches call their activities "holistic health care." Some of these are faddish offshoots that are based on a good concept taken to the extreme, built up as the total answer for all problems, and isolated from the mainstream of care. Unless a health care endeavor is rooted within the total context of the American health care system, it can only remain partial and incomplete care.

In the Wholistic Health Center project, we are demonstrating the merits of some innovative, even radical, departures from the mainstream of traditional American practice. In spite of these revolutionary, although certainly not new, concepts and practices, we have worked very hard to stay rooted within the context of the American health care system. While attempting to offer a unique wholistic approach to health care needs on the primary level, we have also consistently focused on utilizing the best—and there is a lot of strength—in the present system. We have concentrated on coordinating the positive and high-powered technical elements of medicine and offering them to people in a way in which they can utilize their benefits most fully in responsibly caring for themselves and their health.

Although we are perhaps zealots on the merits of the wholistic approach, we are not cultish. Although we deal with a revolutionary concept, we are not revolutionaries. The Wholistic Health Center works within the system. We attempt to find ways of amplifying and coordinating the tremendous resources that the American health care industry has developed, and bring the separate pieces together for the benefit of the patient as a whole person. We offer an unusual model for practicing traditional skills within a slightly revised context, with a wholistic emphasis, utilizing technical information in a person-oriented way. In doing this, we feel that we are offering something more than the sum of the pieces.

Because of our rootedness in the traditional system, it's important to describe the interface between our efforts and the other religious, educational, psychological, and medical resources within our community—an interface that we ourselves take most seriously and have expended a great deal of effort and time cultivating.

## RELATIONSHIP WITH THE MEDICAL COMMUNITY

When describing the Center, one of the first questions the staff is invariably asked is, "What is your relationship with other physicians?" It's an appropriate question.

From the beginning of the project, we have struggled with defining our relationship with other local medical practitioners. Were we to be a full medical service clinic or just a screening center? Were we in competition with local physicians, or a supplementary resource for them—a specialty clinic dealing with stress-related disorders?

## The Past

At first we envisioned that our care would be focused mainly on the "worried well," and we did not emphasize our sickness care services. Indeed, we could not, since we had no full-time physician on the staff. As the concept and the patient load expanded, however, we realized the necessity of offering primary level sickness care as well as preventive services. We began conceptualizing our care as similar to the style of the family practice physician. We began to admit to ourselves as we began to take the medical side of the Center more seriously that we were, in fact, a medical care agency and were to some degree in competition with other local general practice physicians.

As our image of ourselves has matured, we now picture ourselves as perhaps a thirty-fourth specialty—a family practice medical center with special expertise in stress-related, functional forms of illness, rooted in the problems of life-style. As such, we have begun to be seen also by other medical practitioners as an additional health resource to which they refer persons with functional illnesses, who particularly need the wholistic approach for their care. In addition, however, we also maintain a full slate of patients who relate to the Wholistic Health Center as their primary source for medical care.

## The Present

It is possible to describe where we fit into the local medical community by making a distinction between crisis and preventive health care. Every physician is interested in both.

**Figure 10.1    General Practice**

But it's probably safe to say that the ratio between crisis and preventive care distinguishes us from the focus of most practicing physicians. Perhaps 75% of most physicians' patient care and research time falls under the heading of casualty or crisis care, and 25% is preventive (Figure 10.1). The focus of the Wholistic Health Center is about 25% casualty-crisis care, and 75% preventive (Figure 10.2).

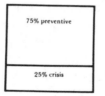

**Figure 10.2    Wholistic Health Center Practice**

Figure 10.1 indicates the kind of medicine practiced by most local physicians in the United States, including those in Hinsdale and Woodridge. Figure 10.2 indicates the kind of medicine we are attempting to offer within the Wholistic Health Centers.

In fact, we have discovered that there is little competition between the Wholistic Health Center and local physicians because local physicians are not wanting to serve nor are they set up to be able to serve the same kinds of preventive care and whole-person needs to which the Wholistic Health Center attempts to respond. Although we both do crisis care and we both do preventive care, our style of offering the care is quite different.

*The Future*

A pertinent question that we hope to answer is, "Can the Wholistic Health Center influence local practitioners to attend more to the preventive care and spend less time in crisis care? Or, can the Wholistic Health Center influence the local medical community to see the great need for the wholistic approach and refer the 50% of their patients with stress-related disease to our 'specialty clinic' for care?"

The answer to the second question is a quiet but definite yes.* Some local physicians are beginning to refer selected patients to the Wholistic Health Center for specific kinds of care unavailable elsewhere. Those who have caught the "flavor" of what we are doing for people have indicated approval of our efforts by utilizing us as part of their medical referral network. Of course, in those cases we do not take over the total responsibility for the care of the referred patient but, instead, offer a whole-person approach, involving the referring physician in the planning, and return the patient to the referring physician for continued supervision of the patient's medical care needs.

For example, one local physician referred to us for counseling a couple that he was treating for a multitude of physical ailments. At one point in the counseling process, the physician chose to spend 30 minutes with the wife, sharing his ideas and advice and listening to her. This encounter made a significant difference in the progress the couple made in counseling. The cooperation and collaboration between the physician and our counselor was a powerful force in helping the couple to keep their marriage relationship creative in spite of some real physical limitations.

Several physicians who had intended to provide health education programs as part of their practice have chosen to

*See Chapter 11, "The Survey of Physicians and Clergy" for details on local providers' response to the Wholistic Health Centers' services.

help us teach our seminars and have referred their patients to our courses. Others have begun to spend more time with patients themselves or have added a counselor/health educator to their staff.

We hope to encourage more of this mutual cooperation and exchange of expertise in the future.

Our status with the University of Illinois Medical School, our advisory group of prominent local physicians, the encouragement of our efforts by the DuPage County Medical Society, the acceptance of our physicians on the staffs of the two local hospitals, and the number of referrals from physicians attest to the fact that we fit successfully into the context of the American medical structure.

## REFERRAL SERVICES

At present a network of agencies and individuals has developed as our "referral system." In addition to contact with the medical community, personal contact also has been made with all of the major mental health, family service, and public health agencies, as well as with the churches in the area. Relationships have been established with the school nurses, psychologists, and counselors.

When we receive a referral from a physician, psychiatrist, school counselor, clergyperson, or nurse, we take seriously our obligation to report back to the individual professional who initiated the referral. The chart of each referred patient is marked with a white sticker with the referring professional's name. At minimum, we call on the phone and report whether the patient did or did not make an appointment, did or did not keep that appointment, is or is not returning for further appointments. At best, when the patient signs a form authorizing our continuing contact with the referring professional, we will regularly report on the specifics of the patient's progress and enlist the support of the referring agent as well as others in "plugging" the patient into a more meaningful, growthful home environment and coordinating the care being offered the patient from various sources. At times, the referring agent has participated with our team in the initial or follow-up planning conference.

The gaps that are sometimes evident in this communication process occur when we do not find out that the patient has been referred. Sometimes during the Initial Health Planning Conference the patient mentions, "Oh, I came because _____ told me to come here." Often, however, patients do not mention that they have been referred. We try to ask, but don't always remember.

## COORDINATION SERVICES

We consider ourselves a short-term primary health care center. Therefore, when individuals need specialized medical services or long-term therapy, we refer them to another local practitioner. Generally, we try to keep our medical or counseling visits with a person to no more than four or six sessions for a single problem. Of course, no firm rule can be made about this. But when it's obvious that therapy over 6-12 months is indicated, we refer people elsewhere. We maintain an up-to-date referral book on providers we have met personally, who work in a specialty area, but who understand and appreciate the value of our wholistic philosophy.

When we refer people to others, we generally remain the "coordinator" of the person's total health care. Too often in the past, we've seen people "fall between the cracks" in the referral process. So we say to the patient, "I know an excellent counselor—here's the reason you should see her/him." We check to make sure that the counselor or physician can respond and will report back to us. We maintain contact with the patient so that while they are receiving treatment outside our Center, they know we are still interested in and in touch with their total health situation.

At times we refer counseling patients to therapy or to educational groups in the community. We may then set up an appointment with them every 4-6 weeks merely for reflection on how the process is going for them.

There is no service we feel is more important than the total coordination of the patient's care. Few professionals or agencies manage to fulfill this coordination of care need, since it's so time consuming and energy draining. Services from all those who have contact with the patient—physician, counselor, schoolteachers, and specialists—must be coordinated. In addition, services have to be linked over time. There should be someone who knows patients through a whole history of personal and family development and can respond to their patterns of life. This coordination function has become central to our care pattern.

Imagine the family whose teenage daughter is hurt in a car accident; it's not difficult to imagine, since the problem occurs frequently. The recuperation is long. School officials and teachers are contacted. The orthopedic specialist says one more bone surgery is necessary for adequate leg repair. The neurologist is continuing to give medication for a head injury, but the parents don't understand why. At home tensions are rising during the long convalescence. The daughter's behavior has changed; she is picking on her younger siblings and is testy with her parents. The parents, with their own measure of guilt feelings, confusion, and anger, are beginning to fight with each other. In the words of a young brother, "The whole family is up for grabs."

Can't someone sit down with this family and help coordinate the information and resources that are available to them from so many different sources? Can't someone sit down with them, get a sense of the turmoil in the family, and help them take a look at it all before the lid blows off?

We've learned a lot about taking on this kind of coordination of information and the responsibility for trying to help it all make sense for the family members. This is actually an act of preventive health care, and it's vitally important.

Every time a serious accident or illness is incurred within a family, there are many providers: the regular physician, specialists, school personnel, perhaps public health people, law enforcement officers, the hospital, employers, and countless others involved in the trauma. Since usually no one has the time to coordinate the care, the family or individual who is already in pain is usually left with the job of making sense of it all as best as he/she can. The Wholistic Health Center, as often as possible, attempts to offer integration and coordination as a necessary and viable health service.

### RECORD KEEPING: THE PATIENTS' FILES

One of the problems in the internal coordination of patient care from the beginning was how we should organize the patient files. Anyone who has seen the enormous medical records accumulated on some patients' physical problems can sense the added difficulty of including information on diagnosis, treatment, and progress for the social, emotional, and spiritual problems as well as the medical problem.

We needed a system that would help us to make sense of the total array of human health problems that may occur simultaneously—a system that could do this yet remain brief and to the point.

*Problem-Oriented Medical Record*

We use the Problem-Oriented Medical Record (POMR) at the Wholistic Health Centers. This system coordinates well with our philosophy, treatment methodology, and affirmation of patients as adults.

In the POMR system all patient concerns are recorded in a problem list and are given a reference number. Notations are made after each visit about problems that were the focus of attention, using four data classifications for each: Subjective (patients' descriptions); Objective (providers' observations in examination or exploration); Assessment (tentative diagnoses, areas for further exploration or evaluation); and Plans (specific goals, strategies for reaching them, and responsibilities for execution).

The Health Planning Conference is an effective way of gathering a data base for the POMR. During the Conference we can record all of the subjective information in the appropriate place in the chart as patients present their concerns. All team members gather objective data as we observe people during the Conference. We can mutually assess the problems with patients and together formulate a clearly delineated plan that patients understand and agree to. Problems recorded on the problem list are often taken directly from people's responses to the Personal Health Inventory. We tend to use the language our patients use in identifying and describing their problems instead of using professional jargon. We often balance the problem list with a "strengths list." In this way we reaffirm that people are more than a pile of problems. Regardless of their state of health, people have resources they can utilize for more effective functioning.

The compilation of the problem list in the presence of patients helps us to understand patients' perceptions of their own health and their own ability and willingness to do something to change. It is important that both patients and staff members perceive the problem in a similar way. If we see the problem differently, we may set unrealistic goals for treatment. Patients rarely comply with unrealistic treatment plans.

By the time the Conference is over and the treatment process is successfully begun, the POMR gives a comprehensive picture of patients not only in terms of physical problems but also in terms of their life-style and other personal or environmental factors that may influence health. We also have a well-defined, comprehensive treatment plan.

The POMR system is especially valuable when patients are being cared for by two or three different providers within the Center. The healing team can review the problems and the progress in relation to each of the problems, so that the plan is monitored as it is being carried out.

Every staff person, including the secretary, who has direct patient contact, is expected to enter significant events into the chart.

*Confidentiality*

Confidentiality of all information is taken very seriously. Since we have such a large number of professional volunteers working directly in patient care at the Centers, we suggest that no one read any charts or share information unless they are directly involved with the care of that patient. Most of our volunteers and paid staff are patients themselves. We treat the people, problems, and progress information for others as we would want our own handled. No one has liberty to page through the files. The phrase we've learned politely to use is, "I'm not at liberty to discuss it."

## Patient Access to Records

We take the position that the patients "own" the information on their charts. Therefore, we invite them at any time to read through their records and raise any questions or suggest any revisions or corrections that may be necessary. Some people have read their records and found minor errors, which we have corrected. Others have read their records and ask that part of the record be deleted because, "That isn't true about me any more." This act becomes a celebration and affirmation of movement toward health. Most patients do not examine their medical charts extensively, but they do know that the charts are accessible to them if they choose to look at them.

## Humanizing Diagnostic Language (Peterson, 1976)

The patients' access to their own charts has caused us to humanize the way we describe symptoms, diagnoses, and progress; especially in the psychosocial area. Objective clinical categories such as "reactive depression" or "acute anxiety neurosis" are seen by patients as a cold and frightening way to label their pain. We have searched for words that might capture the wholistic dimension of the problem, the life struggle embodied in the pain and, most important, the hope for healing that people need to find in the definition of their problems.

People come to Wholistic Health Centers for an incredibly wide variety of reasons, many of which cannot be described in words. Yet we must be able to symbolize a person's situation in some kind of language so that we can communicate, focus, make decisions, and engage the person in the process of becoming healthy. Our choice of language in describing a person's distress reflects our own perceptions and affects our choice of treatment, especially in light of our commitment to address ourselves to problems of the human spirit.

Believing that all people are ultimately and deeply religious and that all of life has a spiritual dimension, we have sought to incorporate humanistic language into our mutual processes of helping people back to health. This is not simply an effort to replace scientific or psychoanalytic words with humanistic words, but a recognition that at the center of any person (including ourselves) is a spiritual core out of which we make the important decisions about life's directions, human relationships, and physical health.

Karl Menninger described the general inadequacy of strictly scientific language to diagnose illness.

> The great paradox is that the patients who today crowd the physicians' offices and fill the hospital beds suffer, for the most part, from conditions to which no simple labels can be given. Their afflictions do not fall into the classical categories of illness painstakingly delineated by our predecessors. They do not correspond to the paradigms in the textbooks. Established names of diseases often seem not to apply to the forms of illness that people are sick with (Menninger, 1963).

Part of the paradox of which Menninger speaks arises from the absence of humanistic language in traditional diagnosis: diagnostic language ignores people's spiritual core and lacks the sound of human feeling and experience. The term "reactive depression," for instance, does not describe the depth of despair or the ultimate possibilities for new life incorporated in the diagnosis of "grief." Nor does the term "paranoia" reach the meaningfulness of a "loss of trust in life and human relationship." The name that we give to a person's situation and the language we use to talk about that situation, with the person and with staff colleagues, has a powerful effect on the choice of healing activity that we recommend.

There are other, more pragmatic reasons for developing our own language. We need a tool to focus, evaluate, research, and record our professional activity effectively. Few people come to us with a single, well-defined problem; their life situation usually includes several problematic areas. Progress is generally made, however, on one or two problems at a time; this requires an ability to focus on the most immediate problems first. We also need to evaluate the healing process, which again requires that we name what we are treating. Scientific research also requires categorization, not only of our patients' problems, but also of our forms of healing activity.

The terms for which we are searching should incorporate both the depth of a spiritual language and the ambiguity of life experience. The language that we are constructing, then, demands that we address the question, "What goes wrong in the lives of people that threatens their health?" To answer that question, we must incorporate a wholistic language into existing diagnostic categories so we can speak of problems of the human spirit.

We have struggled with ways to accomplish this humanization of diagnostic terminology while maintaining consistency and objectivity in the description. Presently, the categories that are used (along with the traditional medical terminology for physical illnesses), and that often help us to describe an individual patient's problems, include the following.

Problems of the human spirit: grief, guilt, loneliness, isolation, meaninglessness, joylessness, stress, helplessness.

Problems of human emotion: expressive, repressive, toughness (anger, aggression, competition) tenderness (love, warmth, intimacy).

Problems of energy expenditure: time, energy, money, speed, pace, consistency, rhythms, control of self.

Problems of information: wrong information, lack of information, lack of understanding, past learning.

The difficulty with these categories is that they lack specificity. The advantage of the categories is that they force us to view patients' problems from a wholistic perspective and in the context of their whole life environment: past, present, and future.

We find that even patients who are health care providers themselves would rather see humanistic, nontechnical language used to describe their problems. Patients prefer "worried about the future," or "a sense of impending doom," or "feels angry and bitter with most people" to "paranoid tendencies." They prefer "grief over loss of a job" to "reactive depression." They choose "lower back pain related to increased stress in present life situation" over "lower back pain of psychosomatic origin."

The exception for which patients request our use of traditional objective terminology is in the completion of insurance papers for reimbursement. For third-party payment, the Wholistic Health Center staff again fits itself into the traditional health care system and labels the problem in a nonhumanistic way that will result in appropriate reimbursement to patients from their insurance companies.

## SUMMARY

We have worked hard to fit into the traditional health care system and yet be innovative and wholistic in focus.

In relating to the medical providers, local hospitals, pastors, social workers; in our referral patterns, in the coordination of care from various specialists, and in accurate, careful record keeping, we have concentrated on fitting into the system of health care that surrounds us and furnishes us with a variety of specific support activities.

Through our focus on prevention and education, our focus on the whole person, our treatment of patients as responsible adults, our teamwork approach to health planning, the variety of treatment approaches utilized, and our use of diagnostic language, we have attempted to search out and demonstrate some comparatively radical methodologies for the delivery of health care.

Both by being part of the system and by demonstrating the real possibility for change within that system, we hope to challenge that system of which we are a part to become a more humanistic, wholistic, and effective mechanism for the delivery of health care.

## Chapter 11

# DOES THE WHOLISTIC HEALTH CENTER CONCEPT REALLY WORK?

Probably the most critical question concerning any innovative venture is, "How has it been received?" Philosophy and plans are nice, but whether or not they work in practice is the key element governing the potential influence the ideas might have on more orthodox medical practices.

Two sources of information about the effectiveness of the Wholistic Health Center are reported in this chapter: (1) the rate of growth, and (2) the survey research conducted during 1975–1976.

## THE PROCESS OF GROWTH

The demand for services offered at the Wholistic Health Centers has increased at a steady rate over their 4-year history. Correspondingly, the Center's income has risen accordingly. It is a common assumption that it takes 3–5 years for physicians starting out on their own to build their practice to capacity. The growth of the Wholistic Health

Centers reinforces that expectation. For the first 3 years of operation, 2 years with a full-time physician (the first year, local family practice residents staffed the Center a total of 7 hours per week), the Wholistic Health Centers operated at approximately 80% capacity and were 90% self-sufficient. Complete self-sufficiency was reached in the fall of 1977.

Figure 11.1 charts the growth of the Centers. The picture of growth offers one answer to the question, "How has it been received?" by indicating a slow but steady growth rate.

## THE SURVEY RESEARCH

Rarely do experimental projects such as the Wholistic Health Center project have the opportunity for systematic self-evaluation in the early stages of development. An Illinois Regional Medical Programs grant to the University of Illinois at the Medical Center, Chicago, Department of Preventive Medicine and Community Health, provided the Wholistic Health Centers with the unusual opportunity for eliciting patient feedback and obtaining local providers' comments on the impact and efficacy of wholistic health care as practiced by the Centers (Tubesing & Strosahl, 1976).

## THE PATIENT SURVEY

During November and December 1975, 387 patients of the Wholistic Health Centers who were 18 years old and over responded to a 94-item, 30-minute telephone interview conducted independently by the Survey Research Laboratory of the University of Illinois. The results of this survey provided valuable data on patient reception of the Wholistic Health Centers.

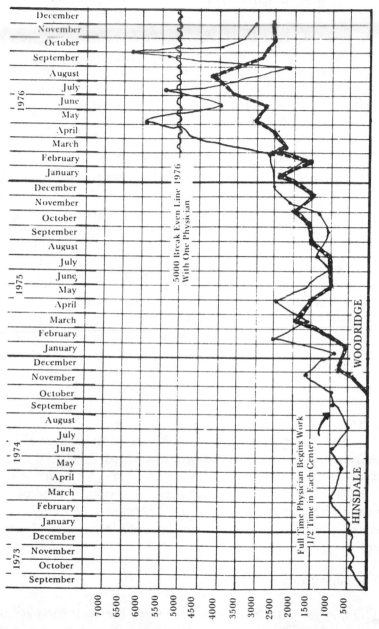

**Figure 11.1  The Income from Patient Fees: *Hinsdale and Woodridge Centers***

189

*The Structure of the Study*

The study sample originally included 673 adults who had been patients at the Wholistic Health Center between July 1973 and September 1975. Decisions were made to limit the sample as follows.

> Patients who were at least 18 years old.
> Patients whose confidentiality would not be jeopardized by participation.
> Only one respondent per household was to be interviewed.

These factors limited the sample to 494 eligible respondents. Of those eligible, 387 (78%) completed telephone interviews. The 22% uncompleted interviews consisted of 18% noncontacts and only 4% refusals. The 18% noncontacts included disconnected phone numbers, wrong numbers, and persons who had moved out of the area or were for some other reason not contactable. The 78% completion rate and the 4% refusal rate are extremely positive and contribute to the reliability of the data collected.

The interviews were conducted by trained Survey Research Laboratory interviewers who used a 94-item questionnaire. Seventy-one of the items (76%) were precoded and 23 (24%) were either field-coded or open-ended questions. The average length of the interview was 30 minutes. Each respondent received an advance letter 3 or 4 days before the first telephone contact.

*The Patient Characteristics*

The majority of the respondents were between the ages of 25 and 44. (Patients under 18 years of age were not surveyed.) Patients who were married comprised 68% of the sample. The male-female ratio was 2:3. The majority of men were employed full-time in white collar occupations. Forty-two percent of the patients had graduated from college, and 30% had at least some graduate training. A majority (58%) had a family income in 1974 of at least $15,000; 18% had an income of $25,000–$50,000. Almost all of the patients were white (99%), and the majority (66%) were Protestant.

Most lived in "nuclear" families (two parents, two children), and 72% owned the single-family home in which they lived. The Center seems to have attracted a smaller proportion of single people in the 18–24 age group and in the over 65 age group than is characteristic of the population of DuPage County, Illinois. However, a higher number of divorced men and women utilized the Wholistic Health Center than would have been expected from DuPage County Census figures.

It can be concluded that the majority of the patients fall into the middle to upper-middle class, and that the patient population is relatively homogeneous.

From the analysis of the sample patient characteristics, it appears that the Wholistic Health Centers are, in fact, attracting persons who are affluent, educated, and have the resources to choose from a variety of health care agencies. The data indicate that the Centers are receiving an affirmative answer to the question, "Will people who have a choice and can pay for their care choose to come to a wholistic care facility located in a church building?"

*Patient Recruitment and Access*

A number of questions designed to gather data on the process of client recruitment and access were asked of the respondents. The basic areas of investigation were: (1) What kind of publicity is most effective?, and (2) How do people make the decision to come to the Wholistic Health Center?

> First Knowledge of Center:
> Eighty-three percent heard of the Center by word-of-mouth sources; mostly from other patients (37%) or from a pastor or church presentation (33%).
>
> Main Attraction to the Center:
> Thirty-eight percent were attracted by wholistic approach.
> Twenty-eight percent were attracted by the reputation of the Center.
> Twenty-one percent came to the Centers because they needed an M.D. or counselor, and either had no M.D. or were dissatisfied.
>
> Prior Pattern of Health Care:
> Most patients had previously established relationships with local medical providers. They chose the Wholistic Health Center from alternatives. In the year prior to their first Wholistic Health Center appointment, 53% had previously gone to a G.P., 13% to a specialist only, 12% to both a G.P. and a specialist, and 10% had no M.D.

A study of the patient recruitment and access questions reveals that personal word-of-mouth publicity, mostly from patient to patient or within local Protestant churches, has been the most effective method of gaining new patients.

Most persons who become patients at the Wholistic Health Centers do so through intentional choice, not by chance. They respond to the Center's philosophy and reputation and choose to come to the Center despite the fact that they have other options for both medical and counseling care. It is clear that the Centers are not, for the most part, attracting the medically disenfranchised.

## Patients' Needs Presented and Treated

PRESENTING SYMPTOMS.    During their first appointment at the Center, 58% of the respondents presented predominantly medical problems, and 42% presented predominantly psychosocial problems. These categories are not mutually exclusive, since the wholistic philosophy of medicine is based on the assumption that most presenting symptoms have both a medical and a psychosocial-spiritual component.

Those patients who initially presented medical complaints were more likely to have moved often, to have lived in the community a shorter time, to have been attracted to the Center because of the convenience, and were less likely to have had a general practice physician than were those who initially presented nonmedical complaints.

MOST SERIOUS PROBLEM TREATED.    Patients who had more than one visit to the Wholistic Health Center were asked to list the most serious medical problem and the most serious nonmedical problem for which they sought treatment at the Center.

The most serious medical problems identified by respondents who listed medical problems included chronic diseases (20%), acute illnesses (21%), physical examination (12%), pain (11%), and other (27%).

The most serious nonmedical problems identified by those respondents who listed nonmedical problems included emotional (51%), marriage and family (39%), and other (10%).

The fact that there is a balance between the psychosocial and medical presenting symptoms is an indication that the Center's patients are responsive to the wholistic approach offered by the Center staff. It appears that patients perceive the multidimensional care of the Centers accurately and are prepared to utilize the wide variety of services available to them.

## Patient Utilization of Wholistic Health Center Services

Most patients had come to the Wholistic Health Centers more than once since their first appointment. Eighteen percent of the respondents had utilized Center services for just one visit; 46% had made two to four visits; 21% had kept five to nine appointments; and 15% had made 10 or more visits to the Center.

Of those patients who came for only one visit, 80% were medical patients, most of whom claimed to be in excellent health at the time of the survey. This group was just as positive in response to the Wholistic Health Center contact as were those patients who came in for more than one visit. It appears that very few patients were disappointed by their contact with the Center.

Of those patients who came for more than one visit, 30% utilized medical care only, 36% counseling only, and 34% both types of service. Those who had one to four visits were more likely to receive medical service, those with five to nine visits were more likely to receive counseling, and those with more than 10 visits were likely to have utilized both kinds of service.

Middle-aged persons were most likely to have utilized both types of service, while the younger and older patients were more likely to come only for counseling services. Both the better educated and the lower-income groups tended to use medical services only.

Forty-six percent of the patient population came to the Center for all their health care needs, while 54% came for only a part of their needs. Those who came only for part of their needs were most typically patients who utilized the counseling and Health Planning Conference services of the Center primarily, but continued the relationship with their personal family physician.

Two-thirds of the patients had participated in an Initial Health Planning Conference (IHPC). The percentage of participation increased during the last year. The IHPC was not practiced before then. Those patients who participated in an IHPC were more likely to utilize both counseling and medical services. They were also more likely to return for more visits to the Center than were those who did not participate in an IHPC.

The Center has maintained a balanced utilization of its care resources by its patients. Approximately one-third came for both medical and counseling care, while the other two-thirds, divided evenly, came for either counseling or medical care.

Generally, the Center staff has been true to its philosophy that the Centers should be short-term, health-related agencies, not long-term therapy and rehabilitation clinics. Most of the patients (46%) have come to the Center two to four times from the time of their first appointment to the time of the survey.

*Patient Evaluation of Services*

*EVALUATION OF WHOLISTIC HEALTH CENTER SERVICES.*    Patients were asked to rate their satisfaction with the services they received from each staff member.

> Ninety percent were satisfied or very satisfied with the physician.
> Eighty-two percent were satisfied or very satisfied with the counselor.
> Ninety-five percent were satisfied or very satisfied with the nurse.

Ninety-five percent were satisfied or very satisfied with
the secretary/receptionist.

The "counseling-care-only" patient was consistently
less satisfied than the "medical only" or "both" patient.
The satisfaction level correlated with the patient's view of
the success of the treatment. In general, the more times
patients had visited the Center, the more likely they were
to be very satisfied.

The patients' satisfaction with volunteer (student-
trainee) counseling was compared with counseling service
rendered by the regular Center staff. There was no significant difference between the rating of the two groups.

The majority of the patients (69%) had recommended
the Wholistic Health Center to someone else.

The satisfaction level and the number of patients referring others is most encouraging. Many patients added additional comments; the most often expressed was, "They
took time with me and really listened to me." This seems
to be an affirmation of the wholistic approach.

*EVALUATION OF THE INITIAL HEALTH PLANNING CONFERENCE.* Of the
67% of patients who experienced the Initial Health Planning Conference, 87% were either satisfied or very satisfied. In general, those who saw their problems in both
medical and counseling areas were the most satisfied.

When asked about their evaluation of specific aspects
of the Initial Health Planning Conference, the patients indicated the following.

Ninety-five percent were satisfied that the wholistic
approach was explained clearly.
Seventy-one percent indicated that the way their problem was defined was helpful.
Eighty-nine percent indicated that the staff took their
ideas seriously.

Eighty-five percent were satisfied or very satisfied with the treatment plan that was developed.

Eighty-four percent indicated that they followed the plan, at least in part.

Seventy-three percent of those who experienced a Health Planning Conference felt that a yearly Planning Conference would be valuable to them.

Surprisingly, 62% of those who were dissatisfied ($N = 29$) with their Initial Conference still indicated that they felt a yearly Health Planning Conference would be valuable to them.

It is obvious that the key mechanism (the IHPC) for the team approach as practiced by the Centers is, for the most part, a successful engagement, teaching, and planning tool. The reception by patients continues to be encouraging.

*IMPACT OF THE WHOLISTIC HEALTH CENTER ON PATIENTS' LIVES.* Patients were asked whether any change had occurred in their lives that they attributed to the Wholistic Health Center. Forty-two percent said "No," and 58% said "Yes."

Those who had visited the Center more often tended to indicate that more change had occurred. After nine visits, however, the likelihood that change had occurred did not increase.

Specific change reported by patients is outlined in Table 11.1.

The efficacy of the short-term, action-oriented approach to helping people take care of themselves and make changes necessary for the improvement and maintenance of their health is confirmed by these data. The fact that the smallest amount of change was reported in health habits indicates the difficulty in promoting change in this area and challenges the staff to concentrate on developing additional strategies for promoting change in health habits.

Table 11.1    Change Due to Contact with WHC
(patient self-report)

|  | Positive (%) | Negative (%) |
|---|---|---|
| Health habits | 43 | 1 |
| Acceptance of self | 78 | 0 |
| Relationships with others | 68 | 1 |
| Family relationships | 67 | 1 |
| Work productivity | 55 | 1 |
| Understanding of personal health | 63 | 0 |
| A sense of personal wholeness | 68 | 0 |

## THE SURVEY OF PHYSICIANS AND CLERGY

During January-March 1976, 267 physicians and 128 clergy from communities served by the Wholistic Health Centers were mailed a 21-item questionnaire designed to assess their knowledge of, reaction to, and utilization of the Wholistic Health Centers for making referrals. The results of this mailed survey are the basis for the discussion of provider acceptance of the Wholistic Health Center project.

### The Structure of the Study

The purpose of the study was to ascertain the providers' knowledge of and response to the Wholistic Health Centers in terms of their evaluation and use of the Centers' services. In addition, it was hoped that an optimal method for communicating the Centers' existence and services to local providers could be ascertained from the survey.

During January and February 1976, the Survey Research Laboratory, under contract with the Wholistic Health Centers, Inc., conducted a survey of clergy and physicians from the southeast quadrant of DuPage County and extreme western Cook County, Illinois. This is roughly the same area from which the majority of patients come.

The physicians in the study were those physicians in

the sampling area who were either registered with the DuPage County Medical Society or on the staff of the La-Grange Community Memorial Hospital. The clergy list was compiled for the same area from community ministerium rolls, the Yellow Pages, church directories, and the memory of prominent local clergy. An attempt was made both for the physicians and clergy to develop a comprehensive list of the providers within the communities selected. Each provider on the final list received the questionnaire. The pretest was administered with a randomly selected sample of 45 physicians and 30 clergy. The final mailing included 267 physicians and 128 clergy.

The pretest questionnaires were mailed on January 2. The questionnaire for the main study was mailed on February 23 with a letter from Dr. Edward Lichter, Chairman and Head of the Department of Preventive Medicine, Abraham Lincoln School of Medicine, University of Illinois at the Medical Center, Chicago. A follow-up reminder, phone call, and a second mailing was sent March 3–12. The responses were cut off on April 12 for tabulation and analysis. Fifty-seven percent of the physicians ($N = 144$) and 76% of the clergy ($N = 96$) returned completed questionnaires. The overall completion rate of 63% for the combined samples is excellent in comparison to most mail surveys with a sample composed of professionals.

*Providers' Characteristics*

While the ages of the two groups were found to be roughly the same, the clergy respondents had practiced in the area for a shorter period of time than the physician respondents. One-half of the physicians practiced primary care; the other half were specialists. One-half of the physicians were in solo practice. Ninety percent of the clergy served congregations. The size of the median congregation was 800 members. Most of the clergy were Protestant and part of multiple-staff ministries. Those clergy who had lived in the community longer and who were either the only staff member of the church or the senior staff member of a larger staff tended to do more counseling.

*Providers' Knowledge of the Centers*

The clergy had greater awareness of the Centers than the physicians. Fewer physicians (24%) than clergy (64%) knew of both Centers, and more physicians (39%) than clergy (10%) had no knowledge of either Center.

The Protestant clergy were significantly more likely to know about the Centers than the Catholic clergy.

Individuals in each professional group were most likely to have heard of the Centers from professional peers (clergy from clergy; physicians from physicians). The Wholistic Health Center staff, the Wholistic Health Center brochure, and newspaper articles were also prime sources of initial knowledge. Many physicians and clergy had heard about the Centers from their patients/parishioners.

Of those who knew of the Centers, 100% of the clergy and 88% of the physicians knew that counseling was available at the Centers, while 90% of the clergy and 79% of the physicians knew that medical care was available. A smaller percentage (84% and 66%) knew that health education programs were available.

The percentage of physicians who know of the Centers is much smaller than that of the clergy. In addition, the younger physicians, who have not been in the community as long, are even less likely to have heard of the Centers than are their older, more well-established colleagues. The Wholistic Health Center staff did not expect the knowledge of the Centers among physicians, however, to be as widespread as the data indicated. The professional peer communication and the communication from patients to their physicians have acquainted many physicians with the existence of the Centers.

Contact with the Wholistic Health Center staff is an important source of knowledge that the Center can influence directly. Other important sources of knowledge (i.e., professional peers and information from patients) cannot be directly controlled by the Center staff.

*Providers' Patterns of Referral*

Four aspects of referral patterns were studied: the percentage of providers making referrals, the reasons for which they made referrals, the satisfaction with the treatment received by referred patients, and reasons for which some providers made no referrals to the Wholistic Health Center. Table 11.2 indicates the referral pattern of the providers surveyed.

Table 11.2    Referral Patterns of Providers

| *Physicians* | *Clergy* |
|---|---|
| **Percent Making Referrals** | |
| 11% of total sample made referrals to the Center(s) | 48% of total sample made referrals |
| 18% who knew of Center(s) made referrals | 54% who knew of Center(s) made referrals |
| **Reasons for Referral** | |
| 22% life change and stress | 20% marriage and family counseling |
| 17% control of health habits | |
| 14% marriage and family counseling | 19% life change and stress |
| 14% personality adjustment | 19% medical treatment |
| **Satisfaction with Treatment of Referrals** | |
| 31% very satisfied | 49% very satisfied |
| 44% satisfied | 29% satisfied |
| 19% not enough information | 18% not enough information |
| **Reasons for not Referring** | |
| 29% no need, no occasion | 3% no need, no occasion |
| 23% not enough information | 26% usually refer elsewhere |
| 22% other, neutral | 23% not enough information |
| 17% other, negative | 0% other, negative |

It seems that the primary care physicians and the pastors of larger churches refer more patients to the Wholistic Health Center. Other factors that increase the likelihood that a provider (physician or clergy) will refer include a provider who is better informed about the Center, has known of the Center longer, and has been in the community less than 5 years. Providers who do refer to the Wholistic Health Center tend to agree with the Center's philosophy.

If referrals are a sign of acceptance, then it appears that a higher percentage of the clergy accept the Wholistic Health Centers than do physicians. However, this observation might be tempered by the fact that physicians have much less knowledge of the Centers than clergy. Getting information to the physicians may be the answer to gaining more acceptance and more referrals.

## SUMMARY

Both the pace of the Centers' growth and the wealth of data obtained through the extensive survey research indicate that the Wholistic Health Centers are successfully translating their philosophy into action, and that the methods developed for applying the philosophy are effective and well received.

The data, of course, also continue to supply the staff with an indication of areas in which the Center can improve, and have offered the staff the opportunity to continue to make "midcourse corrections" based on solid documentation instead of anecdotal feedback. Staff planning workshops, based on these data, have focused on revamping the focus for publicity efforts both to potential patients and local providers. It has caused the staff to establish a program for annual Health Planning Conferences on a regular basis. Other changes have been instituted.

For the most part, however, the research reaffirmed some convictions of the staff (i.e., the Initial Health Planning Conference, although at times a hassle, is worth the effort and volunteer nurses and counselors are perceived by patients just as positively as is the paid staff). The survey has also pinpointed potentially productive areas for more focused and rigorous research, some of which is presently underway.

Is the WHC model transferable to other communities? To other populations? This question cannot be answered without testing the model in various settings. Some of these test settings are presently in the development stages. Without doubt, however, the answer to the question, "Does what you're doing really work?" is indicated clearly from the research analysis.

> We have demonstrated:
> > It really is possible to translate the principles of wholistic medicine into practice.
> > Physicians, clergy-counselors, nurses, and volunteers can deliver quality primary health care together.
> > There are alternatives to the present orthodox system for delivering care.
> > There are positive ways in which some of the problems of the present primary health care system can be effectively addressed.

This is enough on which to continue building wholistic health care efforts at least for now.

*Chapter 12*

# THE FUTURE OF HEALTH CARE

Modern medicine often fails to provide adequate preventive health care for life stress diseases because of the overwhelming demand for crisis care and the failure to take seriously a concept of wholeness in health. Although modern medicine is technically superior to any known throughout history, the neglected aspects of care call for an expansion of health education, an increase in care for the early stages of illness, better coordination of care, and the fostering of support communities for patients experiencing stress-related disease.

## THE WHOLISTIC HEALTH CENTER: A CHALLENGE

The Wholistic Health Center project is one action-oriented research model that proposes an alternative style of care in response to these needs. The project, an innovative experiment in primary care, is in many ways supplemental to the traditional medical care models. It presents a new combination of resources designed to provide a more complete, more economical form of primary care.

What about the future? It appears that the Wholistic Health Center project has a bright future. The first focus for that future is within the three communities presently served. The three permanent, self-supporting Centers, are actively exploring creative methods for helping people to reach unrealized dimensions of wholeness and health. How can even more education and prevention be fostered? What courses will be most helpful to patients? Which tenets of the philosophy have been left dormant? Are families cared for as units? Have any resources for treatment been overlooked? These are the kinds of questions that continually bring the challenge of the future into the present.

Additional future developments will probably include:

*Consumer control.* Some methodology for enlisting patient feedback and ensuring that the consumer's voice is taken seriously in the developing administrative and care policies of the Centers should be implemented. This has been done in the past in an informal way. A system to encourage the local sense of ownership and participation needs to be formalized. Formation of autonomous local boards of directors has already been accomplished.

*Research.* Additional research studying the effectiveness of the variety of care methodologies practiced in the Centers must be undertaken. A study on the cost effectiveness of keeping people well and a solid demonstration of the contention that the Centers do, in fact, keep people well is essential.

*Health care provider's training.* The Centers can become a unique placement site for the training of health care residents and graduate students in primary care, teamwork, prevention, and the wholistic approach. This training will provide students with an optional model for their choice of a professional practice and will help them to experience the resources and insights available from providers in disciplines other than their own.

*Additional "test" Centers.* Centers in a variety of geographical locations, in a variety of settings (hospital, medical clinic, YMCA building, etc.), different kinds of neighborhoods, with other combinations of staffing, and utilizing numerous start-up strategies will add to the growing body of data on the effectiveness and feasibility of this particular model.

But, will the future be filled with a landscape dotted with Wholistic Health Centers at every milepost across the country? No, that's not possible or appropriate, and it's certainly not the goal.

The Wholistic Health Centers stand as visible evidence that small groups of people dedicated to responding to some of the problems in health care, creatively seeking ways to care for whole people, and focusing on health, not disease, can effectively provide a new form of health care delivery. The Centers are evidence that committed people can do a great deal to bring on "The Health Care of the Future: Today." The Wholistic Health Centers raise a challenge to all health care providers, whatever their setting, to find ways of focusing more on prevention than crisis, on a teamwork instead of an isolated approach, and on letting people help each other instead of attempting to provide everything themselves.

But let's leave the story of the Wholistic Health Center project, a young model that is certainly not the only way, but that does indeed speak actively to many of the needs within modern medicine, and go back to completing the examination of the patient, American health care.

## A Prognosis

We began this volume with an examination of medicine (health care) as the patient. We found signs that all is not well. Medical care, due mainly to the spectacular (and laudable) growth of technological expertise, has begun to evidence symptoms of the unbalanced rate of growth: a preoccupation with the body, attention to sickness, not health, a disregard for the context of healing, an infatuation with mechanical manipulation, a lack of coordination, and uncontrolled inflation of costs. The diagnosis revealed that angry consumers, frustrated providers, and the imbalance of the care systems were only surface symptoms of the real problem—that health care has lost sight of health, that people are treated piecemeal instead of as whole persons, and that patients no longer take responsibility for the maintenance of their own health.

The treatment plan called for new concepts of health and health care, as well as for the development of alternative interdisciplinary approaches to the delivery of primary care, focused on education and prevention instead of crisis.

What's the prognosis? Is there any hope for improvement? The answer depends on the patient's behavior. Will the patient follow any of the treatment plans? Will modern health care begin to return to a sense of balance, refocus its efforts on health, and take the whole person seriously? Or will it resist totally and continue with more of the same?

The prognosis is good. The hope for improvement is well-founded, if only the health care system begins to change some of its ways. A crossroads is evident. We can see the problems of health care as a crisis or an opportunity. There's evidence (the Wholistic Health Center, for example) that creative, constructive improvement is still possible within the orthodox health care system. There's evidence that the problems can be seen as a challenge for growth. And there's evidence that change for the better is beginning to occur.

*Signs of Change*

There are signs within the medical system that change is occurring. Medical education, medical research, and medical practices give evidence that they are seeking better, more person-oriented ways to deliver health care. Some of these signs include: the gripes of providers, a positive sign that problems are being felt; the expanding number of new courses in medical ethics; the call for humanizing medical education, and for making problem-solving ability and interpersonal sensitivity criteria for admission into medical school; the arrival of the family practice residency program as an accepted specialty; the the renewed focus on an interdisciplinary approach to the delivery of primary care; the focus on people's responsibility to take care of themselves; and the research emphasis on the "host" for disease instead of on the "invasive agent" that may cause disease.

These forces within the orthodox medical world are strong indications that the future style of medicine will not look exactly like the present system.

The cultural trends also indicate that future health care will combine medical resources in a somewhat different pattern. Cultural signs include: local, state, and federal agencies establishing funding priorities focused on humanizing primary care and developing primary care practitioners; consumer outrage at exorbitant costs, with discourteous and curt treatment (signs that people are standing up for their rights); and the national surge of interest in alternative approaches to the delivery of health care.

The biggest cultural force for change at present, however, is not public concern for the health of our people; instead, it is public concern for the health of our economy.

The cost of paying for the care system we have now will soon destroy our economic stability. We simply cannot keep paying for health care at presently inflating rates. Last year, for instance, General Motors paid more for workers' "fringe benefit" health costs than they did for steel. There are signs that business must, in its own self-defense, look for other ways to deliver more economical health care.

## The Direction for Change

There is widespread interest, arising from felt needs, among both provider and consumer groups in developing alternative models and styles for the delivery of whole-person preventive health care. The time is approaching when the *art* of medicine will again be blended with the *science* of medicine.

All of us, providers and consumers, will in the future focus research on stress—its causes, and ways for coping. We will begin to take responsibility for our own health. We will consider health from a wider viewpoint that includes attention to the whole person. We will focus on education and prevention, not on curing *after* a crisis. We will utilize an interdisciplinary team, not isolated providers.

On the one hand, we need to concern ourselves with retaining the benefits of high-powered, life-saving technology; on the other hand, we must refocus attention on the whole person, on the body's ability to heal itself, and on more person-oriented care. Much of the revolution will occur in our patterns of thought, our ways of thinking about health and disease, the ways we get ourselves sick, and the ways we get well again.

The movement toward a new day in health care is just beginning. It will demand the cooperation of physicians, nurses, counselors, insurance carriers, businesses, unions, hospital administrators, and clergy. It will require the cooperative efforts of most forces within our society.

Whole-person health care is here to stay. There is a revolution in process. It is a revolution that, without disposing of or denying the benefits of technological-scientific medicine, does replace the present mechanical-focused health care with one focused on the total human being and the total context of life. It's a revolution that will begin to return the focus of the health care system appropriately to health and return the responsibility for health to each individual. It will benefit all consumers and providers.

The prognosis is good. Humanistic medicine of this type has been a long time in returning. But it is a force whose time again is ripe, a force that has arrived.

## BRINGING ON THE FUTURE

How can we work to bring the future into the present more rapidly? Much of the control for the pace at which the healing of American health care takes place—for the kind of prognosis we can describe—lies in the hands of the individuals who deliver the care.

Providers' ways of spending time and energy are often governed, not by clear decisions on the most effective style for helping, but by habit. Certain ways to manage an office and care for diseases were learned and are now continued without reflecting on them or questioning them. They are continued simply because they seem to work and because they are comfortable.

It is not the individual provider's task to search for ways in which he/she can revolutionize the health care system. The task for the individual provider is to put all of the habitual ways of managing a practice under scrutiny and analyze whether they are the most effective methods for helping people to become more healthy. The task is for each to consider, within his/her own practice, whether there aren't some ways in which the ability to help people accept responsibility for their health, regain a sense of wholeness, and maintain their health through intelligent planning can be increased. When approached this way, the anger and "sting" is taken out of the revolutionary spirit, and the hard work of figuring out how a more wholistic form of health care can be delivered looms before each of us.

The challenge for all, patients and providers, is to search for what is possible. The challenge is not to open more Wholistic Health Centers, but to utilize the ideas and methodologies embodied in those centers, to adapt them, to restructure them creatively, until each finds some ways in which the principles of the wholistic approach to health care can be translated into action now, within his/her own setting.

## THINGS ANY PROVIDER CAN DO: CHALLENGES AND IDEAS FOR IMPLEMENTATION

The challenge to move toward more wholistic ways for offering health care is a call to break out of old mindsets and broaden the perspective that defines the "territory" and "unwritten rules" of each profession. The old frames that once outlined the boundaries for "proper" care need to be traded in for new, bigger frames that allow room for picturing more of the options. The total human arena, the whole life-style, the feelings, beliefs, fears, and hopes, as well as the family, the job, and the friends, must be considered in the reframing of health care.

The following sections of challenges and ideas are designed to stimulate this creative process, to raise new angles for applying the principles of whole-person health care to a variety of practice settings. They are a collection of possibilities suggested by the Wholistic Health Center model, which could be adapted and applied successfully in any setting.

## The Patient As a Responsible Adult

Central to the philosophy of wholistic medicine is the assumption that the patient is responsible for managing his/her own life and that the patient is capable of participating as an active adult in health care decisions.

### IDEAS AND CHALLENGES FOR IMPLEMENTATION

> The primary method for taking the patient seriously is listening. Why not experiment and listen an extra 3 minutes to each patient? Patients are the certified experts in knowing the symptoms and deciding what they are willing to do for themselves. Listen! Let them tell it.

> Get used to asking patients the question, "Given all these troubles, what is it you need to do to take care of yourself?" See what they say.

> Clarify goals with patients. What problems do they want assistance with? What kinds of help do they want?

> Take 10 minutes to plan with the patient before beginning treatment. Allow the patient to understand the options and to exercise choice over which options are followed. One way of getting at this is to say, "Here are my ideas. Which strikes you as preferable?"

> Practice adult-to-adult politeness. When running late, tell the patient or call the patient ahead of time. Discuss charges directly.

## Care Focused on the Whole Person

The focus on the whole person is essential, but it's not simple. Conscious effort must be made to focus on and raise questions about areas other than one's area of specialty.

*IDEAS AND CHALLENGES FOR IMPLEMENTATION*

Before meeting with the patient, take a deep breath and take 15 seconds to reflect on "What is happening in this person as a total person: Feelings? Relationships? Pace? and so on."

Develop and use a complete life-style (whole-health) questionnaire to replace the usual medical history. Ask people to reflect on their resources and their needs in the various aspects of health: emotional, social, intellectual, and spiritual, as well as physical.

Instead of a "yearly physical examination," adopt a program of annual whole-health checkups and planning conferences.

Learn to ask questions like: "What else is going on in your life right now?" "What do you think is causing this problem?" "*Why* are you sick?" "Why are you sick *now?*" "Why are you sick *with this disease?*" "*How* do you think you can regain your health?"

Look for the creative noninvasive treatment possibilities in other aspects of life and behavior before resorting to medications and surgery. Draw on the strengths in one area of life to help correct weaknesses in another area.

Develop new diagnostic categories that consider the human spirit, life stress, life-style, life pace, and personal belief systems of people. Use them in charting.

Search out the relationship between the "sick" individual and the family context. What in the family is contributing to the illness? What resources for regaining health does the family have to offer?

Utilize the patient's belief system, values, hope, will-power, and other spiritual resources as powerful allies in any kind of treatment plan.

## Attention to the Stress Factors in Disease

There is little doubt that modern life-style and resultant stress is a significant causal factor in the onset of many diseases. Their cure, in order to be more than symptom removal, needs to deal with the underlying stress.

### IDEAS AND CHALLENGES FOR IMPLEMENTATION

Develop and use regularly an inventory that measures the stress "score" of patients. Then help them plan for ways to change behavior patterns to reduce stress.

Look for patterns in people's use of health services. What do the patterns say?

Respect the rhythm in people's life-style. Ask them, "Is this the right time to tackle a behavior change?" "Or to consider surgery?" "Or to take medication as a short-term crisis measure?" The Critical life changes, critical life rhythms, critical life stages are all the result of change. Work at discovering a variety of creative ways to help people deal more constructively with change.

## Prevention and Health Education

Getting to people before they get sick and teaching them how to stay well—this is true *health* care.

### IDEAS AND CHALLENGES FOR IMPLEMENTATION

Estimate your present ratio between crisis care and preventive care. List five ways to increase the percentage of preventive activity in your practice.

Help people plan for the health they desire 10 years in the future. Which daily behaviors multiplied 3650 times will result in greater health? Which will result in sickness? Develop the idea of investing in future health and compounding the interest daily. Start a campaign: "Plan for your health at 60."

Call people on a regular basis (every 6 months or 12 months) and invite them to return for a Health Planning Conference. Make definite return appointments for replanning with everyone.

Offer group educational seminars on health issues that focus on behavior change and personal behavior contracts in addition to information dispensing.

### Teamwork and Coordination of Services

The coordination of various specialized services and the willingness to allow others to offer specialized services instead of doing it by one's self are essential for quality patient care and provider sanity. There's too much information for one person to master.

#### IDEAS AND CHALLENGES FOR IMPLEMENTATION

Within an existing medical practice, involve other people in patient care. Especially focus on involving a nonmedical professional (marriage counselor, social worker, clergy) to join in the diagnosis and treatment planning process. This will make many care options visible to the patient and will provide a rich variety of diagnosis and treatment approaches. Let the patient decide on the treatment plan. Begin regular case study meetings with persons from disciplines other than your own.

Develop a team of resources in Act I of Illness (see Chapter 3) who live with the patient. Call on them and involve them in crisis care and follow-up treatment and prevention programs.

Utilize nurses as health educators for nutrition, baby care, weight control, and so on.

Set up a system for referrals. Know your referral sources. Demand feedback from and involvement with them. Set a future date with a referred patient to "check in" on progress.

Help people make sense of the information they get from various places.

## Fostering Support Communities

Much of ill health relates to isolation. Many people can be supportive and therapeutic to others in need. The "people helping people" process is not the sole domain of professional practitioners.

### IDEAS AND CHALLENGES FOR IMPLEMENTATION

Start a "friends" program for patients, involving volunteer friends who can be therapeutic to patients. Volunteers can fill the gaps and provide care for people who are simply lonely or need someone to listen to them.

Foster the feeling of belonging by inviting patients to group "patient feedback evenings." How about a picnic? A newsletter? Quarterly open forum meetings?

Get a volunteer to locate all local community resources and programs (both official and informal). Keep a card file of these resources up to date. Interest people in experiences such as church groups, special interest groups, community education programs, art classes, self-help groups, and the like, as they need it.

Set up support groups for patients who are no longer in need of crisis care, but who need emotional/social support. Specific focus groups such as cancer groups, weight control groups, stop smoking groups, or general personal support groups for behavioral change are possible.

Visit the family on "their turf" and facilitate their support of one another.

### Develop New Attitudes

None of the challenges will be implemented unless providers take a good look at themselves, challenge themselves to try out new ideas that at first don't feel comfortable, and actively seek feedback from patients. The learning experience could be fun. The following are some guidelines for how to stay alive as a provider without "burning out."

#### IDEAS AND CHALLENGES FOR IMPLEMENTATION

Develop an attitude of *humility* and the willingness to listen and to learn. Listening is not a sign of weakness; it is often therapeutic. A current advertisement for hypertensive medication says, "in the early stages of hypertension    (drug X)    may be the preferred method of treatment." Counter that kind of conditioning by putting a sign on the office wall that reads, "In the early stages of hypertension, *listening* may be the preferred method of treatment."

Instead of trying to act as though you know everything, practice the art of saying, "I don't know, but I will find out." It may be a freeing experience. Utilize other people who have studied the area and do know something you don't.

Learn to accept your limitations. You are a coach, a helper, not an "interrogator-know-it-all-fix-it-person." Practice distinguishing and accepting the boundary between what you can and cannot do for people.

Be a long-range planner. Practice looking way ahead. Consultants (which is what health care providers are) should always try to help people who are locked into their own present dilemmas to see beyond them into the wider perspective.

Learn to take care of yourself. Most likely you treat patients in the same way you treat yourself. If patients were smart they'd say, "When I see how he/she treats himself/herself, then I'll know how I'll be treated." Patients learn more from the nonverbal messages of the model we live than they do by what we say. For many of us, if it's true that we treat others as we treat ourselves, heaven help the others! A "burned out" provider can only dispense help in a mechanical way; people need to be alive and creative and growing and sensitive. Find out what you need to do for yourself in order to stay alive and wholly healthy. Plan ahead. Invest in your own health.

Take care of yourself. Focus on prevention and planning. View your health from all dimensions, not just the physical. Look for creative treatments for yourself.

There's a lot each provider can do in his/her own immediate setting to begin to make the future of whole-person health care a reality today. It's not necessary to get everyone to accept the vision. Not everyone will see the need or the value in the development of a more humanistic, wholistic form of care. But that doesn't really matter. Selling the vision to everyone else is not the relevant task. To be as creative and imaginative as possible, each in our own setting, is our challenge.

*Who Will Do It?*

Who is going to bring this health care of the future into the present? What kind of people are going to play with and test out some of the suggestions in the previous section?

People who are searching are the ones who will implement the future. Medical or nonmedical personnel in helping fields such as counseling, church work, social work, education, and many others, people who will make this vision a reality, are those who:

> Are tired of griping about the system, about patients, about demands on their time, and would rather invest energy seeking alternative ways of helping people solve health problems.
>
> Sense the serious need in themselves that they must find more positive ways of practicing health care or they themselves will "burn out."
>
> Believe that the whole person must be taken seriously no matter what the illness, no matter what their specialty.
>
> Contend that we can no longer accept the definition that health is physical, and that health care is treatment for a body that is no longer working properly.
>
> Want to paint a wider vision and find more creative, less invasive ways for helping people help themselves become more whole.

These are the people who will bring on the future.

## What Is Needed?

Alternative approaches will be tested out simultaneously in numerous contexts by a variety of people across the country. There is a need for communication between persons testing different models and a need for cooperation and a sharing of information. Maybe most important, there is a need for mutual support and encouragement.

*THERE IS GREAT INTEREST.* There is a widespread interest, arising from felt needs, among all helping professions in whole-person health care. Physicians, clergy, nurses, social workers, psychologists, schoolteachers, health administrators, and others are demonstrating interest in rehumanizing personal health care and refocusing on the whole person, prevention, and nonchemical, nonsurgical forms of treatment for disease.

*THERE IS NEED TO GATHER TOGETHER.* While the interest is high, each profession is tempted to look only to itself for recovering whole-person health principles. The approach to wholistic health care, however, by definition demands cooperation and cross-disciplinary vision that can only be promoted as the members of the variety of professions sit down to talk with and learn from each other.

*THERE IS NEED TO DEVELOP NEW MODELS.* Alternative models and styles for health care facilities and individual practitioners are needed to test out additional techniques for offering whole-person preventive health care and to demonstrate the short-term and long-term effectiveness and efficiency of such care.

*THERE IS NEED TO SHARE KNOWLEDGE AND COORDINATE EFFORTS.* Without an openness to approaches somewhat different from one's own, without a sharing of information between professionals in different fields, and without a coordination of services across traditional professional lines of separations, the vision of a more wholistic form of health care will not become reality for more than a few within our society.

*THERE IS NEED TO FIT INTO THE PRESENT HEALTH CARE SYSTEM.* The observation that some "holistic" associations and projects push their own style of care without listening to others and to the exclusion of alternative approaches, and the observation that some of these interest groups are setting themselves up outside of and apart from the established system of health care in our country is disheartening. No movement that works outside of and against the established health care system is likely to have a significant effect on the style of care available to a majority of our population.

*THERE IS NEED TO SPEAK WITH A UNITED VOICE.*     As with the initial stages of any movement whose time is ripe but whose credibility among the bulk of professionals is questionable, the wholistic health movement will be hindered in the "marketing" of its principles if each special interest group goes off on its own tangent and no organizational mechanism for information processing and unified effort is established.

## SUMMARY

We have considered the health care delivery system as a patient. Some diagnoses, some treatments, even a prognosis has been suggested. Certainly, some changes are needed. The patient we've looked at is not dead or even dying, but is assuredly not well at this moment. The recovery, the healing process, has begun. It looks hopeful that health can be recovered in the future.

Will the availability of annual Wholistic Health Planning Conferences, interdisciplinary primary care teams, preventive approaches to health care, and nonchemical methods for treatment be available in the future? Only those of us who live in the present can decide.

We as individuals create our own bodies, our own health, by the decisions we make and the way we live. So also, we create our own system of health care and determine the kinds of expertise, personnel, procedure, and agencies that will be available to us in the future by the kinds of health care on which we focus and in which we invest in the present.

Will the story of the Wholistic Health Center project described in Chapters 5-11 represent more than the simple description of the care procedures of three fairly insignificant, "far out" medical centers? Or will this story, by its vision of what might be possible in medicine if the whole person instead of the individual symptoms were to become the prevailing focus of American health care, prove to be a significant step forward?

The answer to these questions will be determined by people who, responding to the need, set out to build on whole-person care principles. The answer will be determined by people who strike out to create new and as yet unimagined styles for wholistic care. The answer to the question of significance depends on how the concepts are put into action.

We can't say how long it will be until health is recovered. The arrival of the health care of the future depends on the efforts of all of us to reform our system, to rehumanize our concepts, and to rediscover the importance of the whole person.

The arrival of the health care of the future depends on the efforts of all of us to bring the future into today.

# REFERENCES

## Chapter 1

Belsky, Marvin S., and Leonard Gross. *How to choose and use your doctor;
The smart patient's way to a longer healthier life.* New York: Arbor House,
1975, page 235.

Ubell, Earl. "Health behavior change: A political model." *Preventive Medicine*, March 1972, **I** (1–2), 209–221.

Ingelfinger, F. J. Letter to the Editor, *The New England Journal of Medicine*,
February 1976, 442–443.

## Chapter 2

Andreopoulos, Spyros (Editor). *Primary care: Where medicine fails.* New
York: Wiley, 1974, page 56.

## Chapter 3

Andreopoulos, page 31.
Andreopoulos, page 81.
Andreopoulos, page 106.

## Chapter 5

For a detailed discussion of the historical development of the project, see Tubesing, Donald A. *Whole person health care: An idea in evolution.* Hinsdale, Ill.: Society for Wholistic Medicine, 1976.
For further details on the Springfield, Ohio Clinic, see Holinger, Paul C., and Granger E. Westberg. "The parish pastor's finest hour re-visited." *Journal of Religion and Health,* 1975, **14,** 14.

## Chapter 6

For a detailed discussion of the philosophy, see Tubesing, Nancy Loving. *Whole person health care: Philosophical assumptions.* Hinsdale, Ill.: Society for Wholistic Medicine, 1977.

## Chapter 7

Some of the material in this chapter was originally published in Peterson, William M., Donald A. Tubesing, and Nancy Loving Tubesing. *The process of engagement: The initial health planning conference—an interdisciplinary approach to whole person health care.* Hinsdale, Ill.: Society for Wholistic Medicine, 1976. Used with permission.
Holmes, Thomas H., and Richard H. Rahe. "The social readjustment rating scale." *Journal of Psychosomatic Research,* 1967, **11,** 213.

## Chapter 8

From a speech by Dr. Russell Mawby, President of the W. K. Kellogg Foundation, given at the Wholistic Health Center Annual Banquet, Oak Brook, Ill., February 14, 1976.
Some of the material in this chapter is adapted from Peterson, William M., Donald A. Tubesing, and Nancy Loving Tubesing. *The process of engagement: The initial health planning conference—an interdisciplinary approach to whole person health care.* Hinsdale Ill.: Society for Wholistic Medicine, 1976. Used with permission.

## Chapter 10

This section is based on a paper by William M. Peterson, Director,
  Wholistic Health Center, Hinsdale, Ill. (1976) (unpublished).
Menninger, Karl, with Martin Mayman and Paul Pruyser. *The vital balance:
  The life process in mental health and illness.* New York: The Viking Press,
  1963, page 37.

## Chapter 11

For a complete report and analysis of the research, see Tubesing, Donald A., and Sally G. Strosahl. *Wholistic health centers: Survey research
report.* Hinsdale, Ill.: Society for Wholistic Medicine, 1976. The
research was supported in part by Operational contract No. 60,
Illinois Regional Medical Program Department of Health, Education and Welfare, U.S. Government, Edward A. Lichter, Project
Director.

# INDEX*

Acts of illness, 58–65

Allocation of resources, 30; and primary care, 54–66; revision of, 66–73

Alternate health care systems, 29, 86–88, 220–221

American Medical Association (AMA), 28

Anxiety. *See* Stress

Behavior change, 26–27, 59, 62–63, 214–215; and group self-help, 169–170; and health education, 160–164; and HPC, 114, 116, 123–124, 163; pacing of, 118, 146, 214; WHC impact on, 197–198 *See also* Life style; Treatment plans

Beliefs and philosophy of WHC, 100–107, 202–203

Blue Cross-Blue Shield, 28

Body and energy, 83–85

Business, 209; and employee health, 165–166

California "holistic" practitioners, 28

Cancer, 23, 84, 165

Centralization, 54–55, 100

Charts. *See* Records of patients

Churches, 24, 136, 176; pilot clinics, 92–95; relationship to WHC, 89–90, 100–101, 105–106. *See also* Pastoral counselors

Clergy, and health care, 33–34, 44, 51, 57, 69–72, 215; WHC pastors, 135–136; survey of, 198–202

Community programs and volunteers, 104, 106–107

Concepts (American health care), 30, 74–80; changes in, 85, 209, 217; definitions, 78; implementation, 217–218; summary, 86–87

Cooperation. *See* Teamwork

Coordination of services, 23–25, 204, 207; implementation, 215–216, 220–221; and WHC philosophy, 104–105, 177–179

Costs: escalation of, 22, 38, 73, 207–209; GNP percentage on

*The following abbreviations are used in the Index:

    HPC   = Health Planning Conference
    WHC  = Wholistic Health Center
    PHI    = Personal Health Inventory
    POMR = Problem-Oriented Medical Record